Different Loving Too

Real People, Real Lives, Real BDSM

by
Gloria G. Brame, Ph.D.
with William D. Brame

Moons Grove Press
British Columbia, Canada

Different Loving Too:
Real People, Real Lives, Real BDSM

Copyright ©2015 by Dr. Gloria G. Brame with William D. Brame
ISBN-13 978-1-77143-258-0
First Edition

Library and Archives Canada Cataloguing in Publication
Brame, Gloria G., 1955-, author
Different loving too : real people, real lives, real BDSM
/ by Gloria G. Brame with William D. Brame. – First edition.
Issued in print and electronic formats.
ISBN 978-1-77143-258-0 (pbk.).--ISBN 978-1-77143-259-7 (pdf)
Additional cataloguing data available from Library and Archives Canada

Cover artwork credit: Front cover artwork by Ketzl Brame is derived from Naked
man wearing black leather high heels © komargallery | iStockPhoto.com; interior
artwork credit: Handcuffs of love © LostINtrancE | CanStockPhoto.com

Moons Grove Press is an imprint
of CCB Publishing: www.ccbpublishing.com

Moons Grove Press
British Columbia, Canada
www.moonsgrovepress.com

**Note: This book contains frank material on adult topics. It is not
recommended for minors.**

Dedicated to the BDSM Communities for changing the public dialogue about sex and gender, and with gratitude for their support and friendship.

⋛ Contents ⋜

　　19 original interviewees: Alexis deVille, Carter Stevens,
　　Cléo Dubois, Constance-Marie Slater, Dian Hanson, Eve
　　Howard, Fakir Musafar, Gerrie Blum, Baby Glenn, James,
　　Kiri Kelly, Lady Elaina, Laura Antoniou, Mitch Kessler,
　　Morgan Lewis HMQ, Nancy Ava Miller, Robin Young,
　　Sybil Holiday, William Henkin

　　12 first-time interviewees: Chrissy B., Deborah
　　Addington, Guy deBrownsville, Justin Tanis, Karen
　　Kalinowski, Lolita Wolf, Nigel Cross, Patrick Mulcahey,
　　Race Bannon, slave feyrie, slave matt, Stephanie Locke

❧ Introduction ☙

It's 1993, and I'm sitting in the Chief Editor of *Psychology Today's* office with Will Brame, my husband – of now 26 years – and creative collaborator. Our book, *Different Loving*, was about to be released. After much resistance and scoffing from mainstream outlets about reviewing a book on BDSM culture, our publicist Sharyn landed us an in-person meeting with a psychologist who we hoped would take our work seriously.

Sharyn had worked tirelessly to get us on a talk show or nail down the promise of a review in a respected print publication. When a producer from the Phil Donohue show reluctantly agreed to meet us for lunch, they insisted Sharyn be there, presumably to protect them against scary whip-wielding sex perverts. When we showed up dressed in business clothes, the producer admitted she was disappointed by our normal appearance and passed on us. We didn't fit their expectations of social freaks - they didn't know what to do with us.

"The review copies keep disappearing at *The New York Times*," Sharyn said, "but then they act like they are too good to review you. Do you know what someone at the *New York Review* told me? They said it was too heavy to read one-handed!"

We laughed at prudery, false morality, and sexual ignorance but it hurt anyway. After intensively researching the psychiatric, psychological and historical literature about sadomasochistic and fetishistic sex, we knew that most sex theory on paraphilia (so-called abnormal sex) was largely Freudian and distinctly unscientific. When we interviewed psychiatrists who specialized in paraphilia, we quickly realized that most of them still viewed people like us as pathological based solely on the type of sex we liked.

We knew we'd written a book that was worth paying attention to, if only because we had effectively made the first evidence-based case to demonstrate that so-called sexual perversion was an invention of perverted 19th century Victorian men. People who enjoyed exotic acts like whipping, erotic spanking and bondage, or who liked to dress in fetish wear or use clothing to express an internal – rather than immediately visible – identity were not mentally ill, criminal or morally corrupt. They were as normal as anyone else. The problem was that only people like us knew that at the time, while the world continued to believe outdated psychiatric theories.

I knew what to expect when I signed on to write a book about my forbidden sexual identity and people who shared it. I knew it probably spelled the end of my life in the elite New York circles of poets and writers, and that my career as an English professor was over. More than that, I figured there would be lots of people snickering over me, and that it might be harder than ever to be taken seriously by anyone because that was the power of the taint in 1993 when a person like me came out as kinky. I'll save the story of how I came to make the choice to throw chance to the wind in a future memoir. For now, suffice to say, I just knew that someone had to tell the truth about kinky people.

And for one shining moment, sitting in that editor's office, I hoped academic acceptance and interest might help turn the tide of mainstream media censorship. Then the door opened, and a stout and sour woman strode in, sniffing as if there was an unpleasant new smell in her office. She sat behind her desk and stared sternly down her nose at us, shuffling a pile of papers to let us know she was busy. No time for polite conversation.

"How could you call this 'loving?'" she said. "These are sexual aberrations! There's no love involved."

I gripped my husband's hand, and we tried to explain how wrong she was. Since I was still years away from becoming a sexologist, she saw us as BDSM apologists, not credible authorities. Then, just as abruptly, the interview was done and we were dismissed. Maybe she sprayed a little BDSM-room freshener when we left, I don't know.

Twenty-two years later, we can answer all the doubters and anti-BDSM people with authority: BDSM is as loving as any other type of consensual human intimacy. This follow-up volume to our original classic is devoted to that growing body of evidence, and the happy lives, long-term committed relationships, daily realities, and lively communities that make us "Different Lovers."

21st century BDSM

The letter code BDSM was conceived as an umbrella term to cover three related models of kinky relationships. It was hoped that a single, overarching term would allow practitioners to form fellowship over commonality instead of bickering over differences.

Bondage and Discipline (B&D), relationships or role-play involving bondage and punishment scenarios.

Dominance and Submission (D&S), relationships or role-play where one person leads and the other follows, also known as power relationships.

Sadomasochism (SM), the acronym for sadism and masochism is commonly applied today to people who are not interested in romance or power dynamics but enjoy giving or receiving intense sensation.

BDSMers may be any of the above or a combination of the three. They span the gamut, from hedonists who occasionally enjoy pain-play without a power dynamic, to fetishists who crave sensual, power-based play, to lifestylers permanently committed to master/slave relationships. As long as the people feel comfortable describing themselves as BDSMers, they are accepted as BDSMers in the BDSM community.

The term BDSM came into vogue a few years after we wrote *Different Loving*. In the early 1990s, the majority of people we interviewed used D/s or D&S as the least objectionable term.

Using BDSM to describe "What It Is That We Do" (known online as *wiitwd*, a politically correct precursor to BDSM) is largely an Internet phenomenon, as burgeoning communities of kinksters strove to create a common language to communicate more accurately about their likes and dislikes. Self-definition proved critical to forging a new, humanistic language to describe our interactions. Our insistence on not letting psychiatry have the final say about us has, over time, transformed psychiatry. Researchers, medical professionals and psychiatrists now call us BDSMers and not "algolagniacs" (an old psychiatric label for people who enjoyed pain). BDSM is no longer viewed as a symptom of mental illness.

Today's BDSM community is as socially diverse as the general population. The universal values we share are the desire to have kinky sex and to form BDSM relationships. The variety and diversity of BDSM relationships makes it nearly impossible to clinically label relationships, since individuals form their own definitions of what they do and how they do it. Not surprisingly, this same diversity has led to more permeable borders between BDSM and other minority sex communities, including (but not limited to) swingers, polyamorists, trans people, bisexuals, gay men, and lesbians.

21st century BDSM is best understood as a two-headed phenomenon

1. A community of interconnected networks of clubs, parties, and organizations by and for people who identify as BDSMers.

2. BDSM erotic behaviors, spanning a wide range of risk-aware activities such as bondage, spanking, role-play, fetishes, sensation-play and power relationships.

Source: Sex for Grown-Ups, Dr. Gloria Brame

In their effort to analyze BDSM sexuality, activists have helped to shape a larger social dialogue about consensual human sexuality. BDSM expressions – such as "Safe, Sane and Consensual" and "safe words" – have been absorbed into popular culture. BDSM theory and education have led to greater awareness of the importance of informed sexual consent, while BDSM activism has been a driving force in framing sexual diversity as a human right.

But whatever our critics thought about BDSM in 1993, no one, including the pioneers, could have predicted the impact of advances in technology and medicine on sexual diversity.

Three huge shifts no one predicted

1. Internet Communication: linking people together

The Internet has completely transformed the quality of life and social opportunities for kinky people. In 1993, if you didn't live in or near a major metropolitan area, you had no opportunities to meet other kinky people. In 2015, worlds of willing kinky partners are just a few Internet clicks away. In 1993, BDSM looked like a tiny, barely known exotic sexual flavor. In 2015, we know that tens if not hundreds of millions of adults around the globe have some kind of sex kink, enough that they seek out the thousands of specialized pornography and dating sites that cater to esoteric kinks.

2. Internet Consciousness: everyone knows everything

The Internet hasn't just linked BDSMers together, it has also linked us across other lines of sexual orientation and interest. The leaders and founders of Leather Culture were gay men and lesbians and their influence has remained a leading force in the BDSM Community. Similarly, before there was a BDSM community, many heterosexual kinksters attended swing clubs where BDSM toys and games might be found – these days, many in the BDSM world are poly or enjoy group sex or swing events as well. And as all these diverse cultures have morphed, co-supported each other, and forged even stronger bonds online, they have raised universal consciousness about sexual diversity.

Whereas in the 1980s and early 1990s people feared arrest and public shaming if their interests in BDSM were revealed, in a post "two girls, one cup" Internet world, BDSM is not shocking anymore. With global communications, everyone with access has become aware that human sexuality encompasses a seemingly endless array of sexual kinks, fetishes, and entertainingly weird behaviors.

3. Advancements in academic research on human sexuality

In 1991, the research on BDSM was, in a word, lacking. The scholarship through the 1990s still had not moved off the central 19th century assumption that there was something mentally wrong about people who got off on fetish objects, or derived pleasure from painful sensations. It lacked credibility because it lacked replicable evidence – samples were invariably small (as few as four people in some studies); the researchers relied on the people who showed up at their clinics, without interviewing people with the same sexual interests who were not in need of psychological support. Academic research was conducted through a neo-Freudian lens, looking for pathology and presuming to offer cures and treatments (which failed as massively as "conversion" treatment for gays and lesbians). In the last ten to fifteen years, sexual research has broken new ground. There have been numerous reliable studies that have reversed the narrative about the mental health of BDSM people. Studies show that, at the very least, the communication skills required to form a stable, loving BDSM relationship are beneficial to adult mental health and well-being.

Two notable studies showing the benefits of BDSM are:

- "Psychological Characteristics of BDSM Practitioners," published by the Department of Methodology and Statistics, Tilburg University, The Netherlands, which set out to study whether BDSM is associated with psychopathology. The results reported: "favorable psychological characteristics of BDSM practitioners compared with the control group; BDSM practitioners were less neurotic, more extraverted, more open to new experiences, more conscientious, less rejection sensitive, had higher subjective well-being, yet were less agreeable."

- In "Demographic and Psychosocial Features of Participants in Bondage and Discipline, 'Sadomasochism' or Dominance and Submission (BDSM): Data from a National Survey," published by *The Journal of Sexual Medicine*, Vol. 5, Issue 7, July 2008, researchers reported that BDSMers, "were no more likely to have been coerced into sexual activity, and were not significantly more likely to be unhappy or anxious [than the control group]—indeed, men who had engaged in BDSM scored significantly lower on a scale of psychological distress than other men."

When you add up the unprecedented revolution in communication, the unpredictable surge of diversity-positivity as an Internet moral value, and the cumulative effects of evidence-based sex science, you end up with a BDSM world in 2015 that looks very different, inside and out, from the one we began to document in 1991. It seemed like an insurmountable challenge when we started this project to do justice to the vast scope of small changes that have coalesced to so radicalize the understanding of what BDSM genuinely is and how it actually works. The best way to do it, we decided, was to let the Community speak for itself.

ଫ Chapter 1 ଓ
BDSM Then and Now

In 1991, finding enough people willing to be interviewed about BDSM was a challenge for two reasons: most people were in the closet, even within the BDSM communities, keeping their identities secret. We reached out to all the existing BDSM/fetish groups we could find through letters and phone calls, and word of mouth began to spread. Secondly, the Internet was in its infancy, with only a tiny handful of venues bustling with BDSM activity. Nonetheless, through persistence and with the help of interviewees who recommended friends and friends of friends, we were able to reach over 300 people in the course of our research. Of that number, roughly 105 interviews were included in our original manuscript. After editors forced us to whittle the book down by a few hundred pages, we ended up with 89 interviews.

In the intervening years, we lost track of the majority of interviewees. They left the Community, moved to new locations, changed their Internet identities, or took their kinks underground. Several of them passed away, including our original editorial collaborator, Jon Jacobs. Of the 25 original interviewees I was able to locate, a handful declined for personal reasons.

Fortunately, we were able to re-interview 19 of the original participants. A quarter of a century later, many have become lofty icons of BDSM knowledge. To balance and further energize this project, I interviewed an additional twelve people who could speak to different points of view within the Community. A handful are people who should have been included the first time around but didn't make the final edition. Others are somewhat younger activists and private players in long-standing BDSM relationships. I also felt it important to include gay male voices who could speak directly to the gay leather world which has been so vital in articulating and advancing the dialogues about consensual kink and master/slave relationships.

The 31 people we interviewed for this volume represent a smaller but more diverse group of individuals, all of whom have had 20+ years of experience in negotiating and maintaining successful kinky relationships. Together with the additional 150+ people who participated in the "Community Dialogue" portions of this book, we interviewed BDSMers ranging in age from 25 to 85. We selected the best of their commentaries and restructured them into dialogues to provide you with the broadest perspective possible on BDSM life and relationships. These dialogues speak directly to the issues that concern us all: where we came from, who we are, how we live, and how we succeed at forming loving and joyfully consensual BDSM relationships.

- **TIP: Want to know who's who before you read? Flip to the "Who's Who in Different Loving Too" appendix for an annotated list of all 31 interviewees in this book, plus details about the Community Dialogues. You'll find it on page 173.**

NOTE: The names of original interviewees (first interviewed in 1991-92) are identified by asterisks.

Changes in the world of BDSM

The shift in public awareness of and acceptance for BDSM defies ready documentation. Whether it's been the commitment to educating the public by BDSM activists over the years, the intrinsic appeal of fetish wear and creative sex, the friendlier attitude of cops and judges on matters of mutually consensual sex, or if the Internet influence was the critical force in culture change, today's world is very different from the one we wrote about in the original *Different Loving*. You also can't write about BDSM today without addressing the new science on diversity. The Internet itself has been fertile ground for research, and has voluminously demonstrated that human sexuality is not a one-size-fits-all proposition.

Everyone we spoke with acknowledged that the changes in the world of BDSM have been astonishing, unforeseen and unfathomably swift. In 1991, the mostly underground BDSM Scene counted members in the thousands, and grew into underground networks – clubs, advocacy organizations, play spaces and national conventions – which gave BDSMers a sense of security within our world. More often than not, people new to BDSM were mentored into our world by friends or lovers. Word of mouth was the most powerful networking technique. The BDSM community was small enough that you were never more than 2 or 3 kinky friends away from someone who could give you the scoop on someone you wanted to play with or who could help you figure out if they were safe enough, sane enough, and had the right toys.

Similarly, in all the BDSM underground networks of the 1960s - 1990s, leaders were known quantities, often long-time activists and players, and it was easy to vet them to be sure they were truthful about their experience. This created a profound sense of warmth and kinship at clubs and events. The big danger then was stranger SM – going home with someone no one could vouch for.

The 21st century "Community" is a global phenomenon, where anyone with access to the Internet can find a kinky hook-up. The membership numbers on the two most prominent BDSM dating sites are revealing. FetLife (short for FetishLife, or fetlife.com), a BDSM-community-oriented dating site, claims over 3.5 million members worldwide, people who are either already involved in BDSM or are looking for people who will do BDSM with them. Recon Leather Dating (recon.com) similarly claims millions of gay and bisexual members around the globe.

The BDSM world of today mirrors Internet culture. It is fragmented, specialized, and less of a consolidated community than a multi-tentacled socio-sexual Cthulhu. Sheer numbers, and the rapid influx of unknown entities, make vouching and vetting impossible outside of long-established groups and cliques. Leaders appear and vanish, preda-tors and narcissists install themselves as experienced dominants, and financial scandals have rocked trusted major BDSM organizations. There is no telling if people today will even read a book or learn what Safe, Sane, Consensual means before exploring BDSM sex. The popular-ity of BDSM conventions and educational outreach programs is declin-ing as the demand for online dating and immediate gratification rises.

Ironically, as big as today's BDSM community seems, the number of kinky people who attend events and clubs are an ever-shrinking percent of the number of adults who do BDSM privately with partners or solo at home. Someone is buying all those flimsy whips and fluffy bondage cuffs, and it turns out to be tens of millions of people who never show up at events or post profiles online.

In 2015, deluxe sex toy maker, Lelo, tried to gauge general attitudes towards BDSM among their consumer base by conducting an online marketing survey. They counted roughly 1,100 participants, average age 18-25, and reported that "three quarters of respondents have tried BDSM in one form or another," with 80% of respondents claiming "al-ways wanted to try it" as their main reason for doing BDSM (as op-posed to reading a book or being initiated by a friend). 90% of all re-spondents said they see BDSM behaviors as part of a normal, healthy sex life. The data may not be scientific but nonetheless speak volumes to the growing acceptance of BDSM.

What BDSMers think about BDSM today

We asked our core group of interviewees how they felt about the BDSM world as it exists today. Their opinions encompass the current thinking trends on the BDSM community. (Note: Original interviewees have an asterisk next to their names.)

Everyone is keenly aware that the Community has changed enormously. Some people find the changes off-putting and worry about troubling new trends. Your thoughts?

*William Henkin From what I see, from what I learn from friends, and from what I hear from clients, associates, and other sources, it seems that the scene I knew is utterly gone. To a large extent I think the community has become widely democratized in a way we could not have imagined as recently as, let us say, 1990, and I attribute the wholesale dissemination of its information to the rise of personal computers and the astounding growth of the net.

I find this expansion of knowledge to be an excellent occurrence, in general, but like all excellent occurrences it has its downsides. As if the community had been a secret society that for some reason chose to open its doors to all, more people have more access to more information all the time, which I see as a good thing. At the same time, and almost as a corollary, fewer people have the hands-on relational experience that pushes them to translate their information into knowledge, and even if the number of people capable of transforming knowledge into wisdom has remained constant – which, who knows? – the proportion seems to me to have diminished, which I see as very broadly sad and unfortunate.

I don't mean that the careful training that once went into earning your leathers does not still occur, or that the delicate nuances of play are no longer obtained, but rather that they are no longer de rigueur. The Community has dissipated so that an alarming number of people now hang out their shingles as Dom/mes, Masters, Mistresses, slaves, submissives, and so forth without – to my mind – adequate supervision and without much investigation into what the terms mean, or how and where they are aptly applied. A perusal of some of FetLife's 50,000 groups bears me out: a disturbing number of people assume they know answers to questions they do not even seem to understand.

Deborah Addington When I was first introduced, I had to be introduced, literally. People relied on each other for community building. There was no way to locate an event and simply decide to show up. That isn't generally true anymore; you get on the Internet and you can find something kinky to do pretty much any day of the week. In the process of becoming more visible and accessible – which has its benefits – we've lost a facet of personal connectivity as an essential component of community building. The new world of BDSM is much broader. It includes everyone, from the weekend pervert to the utterly precisely refined specialized practitioner to Master Dragonbreath who buys a whip and announces he's a Gorean. While we have the benefit of access to a broader range of people and activities, we don't have the same types of models for building community because the growth has happened so quickly. We've done an amazingly effective job teaching others how to do, as in technique and appearance, but the absence of core, connected communities has meant that we've not done so well with educating how to be.

*Carter Stevens Today's scene is much bigger and yet in some ways much smaller. Thousands maybe even millions are part of the online scene but 90% of them wouldn't know one end of a riding crop from the other. The "real life" scene has splintered into many factions and cliques that all look down on anyone not part of their clique. When we started our Weekend long BDSM resort parties in the Poconos there wasn't really anyone else who was doing what we did. Nowadays there is an S&M party/event someplace every weekend it seems.

*Constance-Marie Slater What I find is that people do not understand SM. They've lost sight of the pleasures of it. They're not using power over other people in controlled ways, but in dangerous ways. There used to be respect, and there was an understanding among partners that we were doing it for sensuality, and using safe words and rules to keep it healthy. Now people are doing it as if it's a fad, and I find that unsettling.

Karen Kalinowski Leather, tattooing, owning a sex toy/flogger/blindfold in the bedroom all seem fairly mainstream now. Magazines oriented to all gender orientations regularly discuss sex and kink more openly. People who thought of themselves as being really abnormal realized that lots of people shared their enthusiasm for something a little more "spicy."

The downside to this is the number of people on social media/at events who now call themselves "Master/Sir/Mistress" without ever having really earned the right to that title. Previously, there was more ritual around "earning your stripes." That still happens in some places but overall there doesn't seem to be the same interest in mentoring people as there was previously. People feel like they can learn everything from a book or by watching online porn/kink. The code of honor we once believed necessary in our communities seems to be vanishing. People don't hold the same respect for community elders who have gone before them as before. This can make it very difficult when choosing play partners because it's hard to know what level of expertise their potential playmate might have. There have been a few reported injuries and casualties lately. When proper education occurs via mentoring, these accidents are less likely to happen.

*Morgan Lewis HMQ It's nothing like it used to be. It's the computer now, with all these hussies who think it's all about extracting money from men. They think they can hurt a guy, or kick him down, and that's what domination is about. Loving SM is not out there unless you came from the old school. You have to be careful who you follow and listen to. There are people out there in real life to say positive things about BDSM. They aren't there to rip you off, like so many of the women online.

I went to a prodom's website, a woman who was so beautiful, but when I got there, she had photos of her with her legs spread. That isn't dominant. That's just sleazy. How are you going to draw men to you looking so cheap? People think everything is on Google; but no, you cannot Google how to genuinely be dominant.

I'm not a snob. I might be a big slut in bed, but I wouldn't put it out in public. I can't get women to understand that if you're going to be dominant then you have to show it – be a lady, be in charge of yourself so men will want to come to you. There's nothing more intriguing than a woman who draws your eyes just by walking across the room. All of that is gone when there are graphic images with price tags behind them. It takes away all the beauty, all the sincerity, all the mystery out of BDSM.

*Lady Elaina When I was coming up in the scene, when diseases were much less a factor, play was generally a prelude to sex. Now, it is often completely separate. I believe that is because the younger folks grew up in such a different sexual reality, that it was just a lot safer to play and keep sex as a separate item.

I do very little public BDSM these days, having seen play in the scene move to steadily more violent and brutal play. I get upset watching a lot of the stuff I see out there, so I rarely visit play venues now. I have a large, well-equipped and elegant dungeon space in my basement, so I play at home. I am a sensual eroticist. I understand the desire for endorphins, dopamine and serotonin. I can produce that in my bottoms, subs and slaves without the brutality that seems to have become so common. I founded and run two educational groups here in South Jersey near Philly, the South Jersey Power Exchange for BDSM education and MAsT:Edgewater Park, because I have seen the loving eroticism go out of the play I see today. I see cruelty and anger purged on the sub. I see Dominants taking all their subs' money, and I see a large percentage of inelegant play that is based upon beating the crap out of the sub like cavemen. We can do better than that. Much better.

Some of our interviewees feel a bit alienated by the changes in BDSM mores.

*Laura Antoniou I am still active in BDSM by default because I'm a writer and a speaker and teach classes. But I join no clubs, donate hardly any money, and don't raise funds for organizations any more. I'm tired of seeing my money get stolen by people, especially people I've known for years. I'm also tired of being poor. If people want to give me money for a good cause, I can tell them all about how much more I will write if I won't have to get a job selling lattes.

*Alexis deVille It is a bit confusing. A lot of younger Club people dress for it but do not partake, which has caused me a bit of embarrassment! A lot of young people wear the badge, but it's more like a hobby. I've run repeatedly into that, especially in the New York dance clubs. You have to be careful in the clubs because now a lot of people wear the clothes but have no idea. It's strictly a fashion statement for them. The days are over when you could recognize leather or fetish people by their outfits.

*Baby Glenn I think BDSM is coalescing in part with help from the Internet, but as it does so subgroups within the Community seem to be taking the position that SOME interests are acceptable and others are not. It's fragmenting the Community into factions. It's odd and disheartening to see members of a community that at one time was universally condemned now condemning one another based on judgments of specific fetishes or BDSM practices.

*Gerrie Blum In 1995 I had the opportunity to become the publisher of The SandMUtopian Guardian, a factual, useful journal for BDSM people of all persuasions. For five years we solicited and published articles of interest to a variety of men and women, highlighting techniques, relationships and the scenes across the country. However, as the 21st century dawned, we found that the quality and frequency of the contributions were declining.

These days I am not active in the club and organization scene. I have "aged out" as the scene has broadened and gotten younger in average age. And, a "time out" a few years ago to deal with cancer left me somewhat out of energy and out of touch. But I still come to the shop every day and enjoy keeping in touch with BDSMers by phone and email.

*Mitch Kessler What very little I see of today's BDSM scene comes to me through requests for contributions to event silent auctions... and the occasional dip into kinknet.com. Having lost most of my looks, and almost all of my taste for conflict, judgment, and lecturing others, I've been out of circulation for over ten years. The BDSM craft work, with its attendant vicarious involvement in other people's kinks, continues to engage me though.

The BDSM community was always a mixed bag for trans people, who have at times felt isolated, ignored or judged.

Justin Tanis More people are aware of trans men and women in the community than before and I think (but am not positive) this has resulted in better treatment. I think there are still some very transphobic elements of the community or men who think that putting down trans men will help assert their masculinity/gayness. I've had a few people not want to be with me because I'm a trans man but by and large, I don't think I've experienced a lot of transphobia in the Community. Or maybe I've done enough advocacy that I just ignore people who are jerks.

Chrissy B. Trans women have always been a part of the scene, but our niche 25 years ago was a lot smaller, probably because there were fewer of us who were "out" enough to get to know people. At the moment we're the flavor of the month, and as a result there's been exponential growth in the population who are visible and available. While there's still some residual hostility between some in the LG segment and the BT segment in the LGBT rainbow, that, too, seems to be subsiding.

For others, the changes feel positive and have fit seamlessly into their lives.

*Nancy Ava Miller I think what's happened since the first volume of *Different Loving* is amazing! When I started out, there was nothing. I saw my mission. I attended meetings at TES, and when I returned to New Mexico in 1986, I started PEP. Then I went to Washington and started PEP there, a group which later became The Black Rose. Now, with the Internet, there are groups in almost every little town in America you could go to. It was so different when I was traveling the country and setting up groups where I could.

I feel that my job is obsolete now. In the old days, I might have done 3 PEP meetings a week but it was all PEP. Nowadays, on any given week in Albuquerque there are 5 or 6 events that people could attend. There are poly groups and BDSM ones. There is even a wet munch (lunch social where alcohol is served). It meets at the Press Club and you can buy drinks. That's another change, because in the old days, BDSM meets were strictly alcohol-free.

I still attend Club Femme and Alternative Erotic Lifestyles (AEL), led by Stan Alexander, who I really respect. I love talking about BDSM and hearing lectures. I'm not much of a party person. I find it disconcerting to be in a big play space with people who don't know each other. So even when I do go, I end up schmoozing and noshing and never making it into the dungeon space.

It seemed like we had a much older crowd in the past, people mainly aged 40s-70s. In those days, someone in their 30s were practically like babies. Now you see lots of college-aged kids. They're open about their interests. They occasionally bring their vanilla partners along just to meet kinky people. People are so much more educated today. They know so much more. And OMG – do you remember how hard it was to get women to attend events? Nowadays, it's 50/50 men and women, and everyone is out and happy. There are lots of married couples involved now. It's incredible.

*Eve Howard Spanking parties have become one big, international floating convention, with the half-dorky/half-hip spanking jet set planning most of their vacations around them. We held our first event of this nature in 1991 and hosted our 25th party in Vegas this Labor Day Weekend, 2015.

With ages ranging from the barely legal to the barely ambulatory, the live social end of the scene is remarkably diverse. The range of available play options is correspondingly expansive, encompassing everything from the so-called "Littles" (age-players, diaper fetishists, and Adult Babies) with their crayons and pinafores getting birthday paddlings, to the full blown floggings of double-dildoed slave sluts, with plenty of room in the middle for traditional home and school discipline, institutional discipline, clinical discipline, romantic spanking, erotic spanking, and of course, the all-time favorite, spanking as sexual foreplay.

That people continue to support scene clichés is interesting to me. I've often poked fun at such things in my Shadow Lane books. For example, the tradition of telling newbie submissives that they are "not real submissives" unless they do such and such and allow others to make decisions for them. A lot of my stories revolve around girls who decide not to drink that Kool-Aid.

*Robin Young I must give a shout out to FetLife.com, a really successful (in my experience) online social network for the BDSM community. FetLife has given me and many friends a place to share and enjoy each other's creative sexualities to a degree not previously possible. I am very grateful for its existence.

More generally, my wife and I have a coterie of kinky acquaintances here in Seattle, for whom we are very grateful. I do not participate as much in the public BDSM community, mainly for lack of time, but also because I find smaller and more selective groups to be easier to get to know, and more fulfilling.

Nigel Cross One thing I've discovered in 30 years' worth of interactions with other BDSMers (both men and women) is that despite the distinct desire to want to live this life in the open, there are too many hurdles against doing so, both in society and social interactions. It used to bother me so much that people are ashamed of being what makes them most comfortable, when they should be overjoyed at being exactly what they've always wanted to be. Hanging out in online BDSM social circles makes life so much more enjoyable, especially since I live in a conservative community that has zero BDSM activity or awareness.

*Kiri Kelly I am pleased to see so many events taking place, such as the Bash in Orlando, Fetcon, Beyond Leather, and other lifestyle conventions. I think that the classes they offer are valuable, and are especially important for those new to the scene. There can be a danger aspect to a variety of fetishes and I believe it is important to have proper instruction from those who are knowledgeable before risking the safety of a loved one.

Other than getting together with our small community of friends, my wife and I are part of a local group of women into BDSM and we periodically gather at different members' homes for fellowship and assorted BDSM themed parties. I do wish that there were more local munches. There seems to be a lack of venue space to gather the local community and we are forced to have smaller parties at homes with a group of friends, instead of being able to interact with the greater community.

Long-standing BDSM educators and activists have remained committed to keeping education authentic and accommodating the changes in culture.

*Cléo Dubois Today is not yesterday! I don't want to go into the often difficult pioneer/settler dynamic that arises in all communities. Everything changes. I am glad that kink is not pathologised like it used to be. We all worked on that very hard. We saw leather shift to BDSM, now kink and perhaps kink lite. But, I am in San Francisco, still the capital of sexual freedom and diversity. I support my community dungeon, I teach classes, present at local and national leather conferences. I had the honor in November 2014 to be inducted in the Society of Janus Hall of Fame and be part of their 40-year celebration. As LGBTQ and Kinky, we have marched a long time for acceptance, not in an effort to lose our identity, but to reach out to a much larger group.

What matters to me is passing on awareness of the roots of our practices, the importance of integrity, and the potential for sacred connection in our kinky sexuality. That work is not over and I love the work.

*Fakir Musafar I think it's fading, changing, morphing. It's more inclusive of people who wouldn't be in the scene years ago. For a long time we had a gay scene and a hetero scene, and now that distinction is fading too. They are very aware of how much the scene has changed.

What was once private small communities have gone mainstream. It is important to honor the past and the pioneers – a lot of people playing around don't bother. They lose the spirit, the energy, and all the good we built. Still, it is our duty in continuing to pass the message along. Not to throw up my hands in despair but to go into these groups and educate them on what really has power and spirit.

If older people really want to be of service they should go out and help guide the new communities. There are a lot of people who need mentors and teachers because they have lost their way. I do my best, and play my role wherever I can effect positive change. That's why I am so active in training people, so they can go out and continue to put forth information and education.

Race Bannon The scene I entered in the 70s was a much simpler thing to navigate. It seemed less prone to dramatic upheavals or disagreements. We didn't have social media so we couldn't amplify a few loud disgruntled voices and make them seem like a majority opinion. It was just simpler and far more sexual a scene than it is today.

Once upon a time the BDSM scene was a fairly monolithic thing. Most of us thought similarly, played and socialized mostly within our own demographic, attended the same few events, belonged to a fairly small number of clubs, and so on. Then, starting in the 80s, there was an effort to blend the gay, lesbian, heterosexual and other BDSM camps into a unified pansexual community. To some extent that's succeeded, but at a price. Today, I'm seeing some balancing taking place with BDSMers deciding that sometimes they want to blend and other times they want to be with their own kind. The same together/separate struggles are happening in clubs, organizations, bars, leather contests and online sites. Anywhere we've blended there are signs that while some want to retain the blending in many instances they also want a clear separation in other instances. I think we need to honor that or it's going to decimate the organized BDSM scene.

I think the scene is bigger than ever, more educated than ever, with more events than ever, and also at the same time more fractured than ever. I'm not really sure whether the fractures are bad or just evolutionary. Ultimately I think the BDSM scene is better than ever. We have our bumps and bruises (some of them welcome), but somehow most of us seem to get along and figure out how to have pretty damn good kinky lives.

Lolita Wolf Working in a BDSM boutique like Purple Passion (NYC), I find a lot of people don't know about BDSM education, and won't have anything to do with it. Some people are learners and some aren't. You can't cram education down people's throats. I get non-BDSMers wandering into the shop every day, looking to buy an anal toy without knowing any of the basics of anal sex. They have a partner who wants to try it and they are ready to do it, even though they don't know how to safely put something up another person's butt. Some of them don't even want to hear the long explanation about the safest ways to do it.

Informed, adult consent was something we educators kept hammering on: BDSM must be mutually consensual. Now that phrase shows up in the media all the time. It means that people in their 20s are now hyper-aware of consent, far beyond what we were. Unfortunately, they can be so hyper-aware that it creates problems because they want to negotiate every act and get explicit consent every step of the way. This means intense negotiations on what you can and cannot do. This over-negotiating is too much for me. Instead, I have become really careful about who I play with. I make sure that I form relationships with people who are on the same page as me, who allow me some leeway and think that it's hot if I'm spontaneous or surprise them. I now limit myself to people who really love these things and trust that I'm safe.

In some ways, BDSM has been watered down. AIDS came and the safe sex laws in NY changed what we were allowed to do. We had to separate our sex from our BDSM. I think it's one of the reasons sex is still separated from BDSM. I fear I had a hand in promoting that and regret it. People take things too seriously now, and don't see that it's just for erotic fun. I'm very often irreverent about the over-seriousness, or the idea that there are fixed rules on what BDSM is supposed to be.

Some of the older BDSMers say, "Oh, younger people, they don't care about our history and the way we did things." I accept it. I think it's okay. They aren't doing it the way we did it – they're doing some things better, and they bring a different energy to it. There's a lot more information out there than when I started. There are books and videos, there's Kink Academy, there are educational events in almost every city. Everything is so much more accessible and the toys are so much nicer too!

Patrick Mulcahey I was director of a dedicated education program, the San Francisco Leathermen's Discussion Group (SFLDG). Our only demo or technique offerings were presentations by great players intended less to "teach" than to inspire. There's nothing like learning from great players – what they have is more than "skills" – but that's not always available, and not ever to some folks. The compensating migration of kink into classrooms is mostly dispiriting to me.

We are always sounding alarms about kink information on the Internet: "You can't learn needle play online!" True enough – but you almost can. And most of what we do is even less complicated. It makes me crazy to see the beauty and power of what we do reduced to a revolving-door dozen of Safety First lectures. We need one-on-one mentorship back. Certainly we have the numbers for it. It's already started in some places: SFLDG has had a thriving mentorship program for the past several years.

It would be nice if our larger events would facilitate that kind of interaction, instead of sending out blanket solicitations to fill workshop slots. Newcomers look at conference workshop schedules and think, "So this is what I have to know?" The kind of education I think is indispensable is what we're doing right here: telling our stories. Who we were. Who we became. What changed us. What led us, and where.

*Sybil Holiday I have watched the leather community(ies) change so much since 1980 when I got involved. I don't know if, 20 years from now, there will be even a "leather" community. It's possible "leather" will become a subset of "kink."

Leather and SM were intricately melded when I got involved. They aren't anymore. That's because people's kink interests are actually much broader than leather. Leather has become a choice now; a thing that people do because they are interested in that particular structure and tradition. And SM has become something that some do without any D/s or power structure at all; it's simply intense sensation. This is a good thing because when I got involved we were all Tops, bottoms, and then Masters, Mistresses and slaves; there were no bondage enthusiasts, or those who were simply masochistic. It was harder for bottoms to get their needs met directly.

But every subculture changes when it starts to become popular. BDSM has had so much exposure in the last three decades, it's inevitable that kink culture would bleed into pop culture, like Madonna's photo book *Sex* in 1992, or more recently that atrociously written and misinformed book *Fifty Shades of Grey*. I don't see any of it as inherently good or bad, it's just how life is. Life changes. It's up to us to figure out how to live with it, talk about it, and be honest about it.

Guy deBrownsville When I first came into this world, rope was something that a few people did and did well, but which most people weren't into. Today, rope-play has become almost a cult with some. The same was true with "edge play" for a while, where people tried to be edgier than the next person to show how hardcore they were.

I've also noticed divisions deepening. Some people in the 35 and younger crowd (The Next Generation or "TNG") feel a genuine disdain for BDSM elders. I've heard some pretty nasty comments being hurled toward older BDSM practitioners. Conversely, I've seen quite a few older ones, some who have adopted names like "TOG" (The Older Generation) or "COP" (Creepy Old People), rail incessantly against "the lack of respect these young people are showing." So it cuts both ways. Politics divide people. Similarly, while race issues have always been just below the surface of culture, current events make race relations another area for divisiveness within the BDSM world today.

The focus on consent violations is another double edged sword. It is very important to make sure that everyone feels safe to practice the things that we enjoy. At the same time, it is difficult to imagine a way to adequately provide a means for due process in the case of accusations. How can we be fair about handling these problems as a community? The discussion has led to a great deal of debate and polarization.

On a more positive note, the discussion of BDSM has become more open and more people are asking questions and opening themselves up to exploration. There is more information out there, so BDSM is not as hidden and forbidden as it once was. Younger people are not as afraid to display their involvement as they once were and the social stigma is not as high as it was even a few years ago. We are nowhere near Nirvana, but we have made significant progress.

As a media representative for The Eulenspiegel Society [*founded in New York in 1971, TES is the oldest and largest educational/peer support group for BDSMers in the world--ed.*], I participated in far more positive reporting from mainstream outlets than ever before and have seen more unbiased educational information aired by media than the sensationalism that was the norm in the past. The bias against us still exists in many quarters, but people are getting a more balanced view now on BDSM, and that's a good thing.

Finally, a prominent publisher weighs in with a broader social perspective on the changes.

*Dian Hanson I've seen Kim Kardashian in a rubber dress, and a whip cracking dominant in a pistachio commercial, but I don't see very much fetishwear here in LA otherwise, and certainly not as much as in 'the '90s, when there were so many fetish photographers, fetish books and magazines driving the popularity. TASCHEN published Eric Kroll's *Fetish Girls* in 1995 and it was a big seller for the company, but we've now stopped publishing fetish titles because demand has declined for images of women in dominance gear. We are about to publish a 20th anniversary edition of Richard Kern's *New York Girls*, which has a strong bondage and post-punk element and I'll be very interested to see the response.

This doesn't mean there are fewer dominant or submissive people, but maybe that they've learned the trappings are just fashion and meaningless. As far as the vanilla public's understanding: *Fifty Shades of Grey* (and its sequels) seemed to come as a big surprise. "You mean many women enjoy bondage and submissive play?" as if there had been no headway in educating the public about alternative forms of sexuality in the last 20 years. And what could be more common than female submissive fantasy? It hardly even qualifies as alternative, yet the media expressed shock, and no small amount of titillation, and every interview I did for six months asked me to analyze this "modern phenomenon." I told them it's always been the most common female fantasy and kept hearing back, "but women today are liberated and want respect and power," as if the bedroom and the boardroom were one. And we still have far more women than men claiming to be shoe fetishists, just because they buy too many pairs, with no understanding of what true fetishism entails. Tell them that if they're truly shoe fetishists they'll be sexually aroused by shoes and require them to reach orgasm and you get choruses of "Gross!" So maybe the increased casual use of the word "fetish" has made things worse for real fetishists, made them more marginalized, because the word's sexual connotation has been lost in common usage.

On the other hand, the Internet has made it easier for young people to research every aspect of their sexuality, to put names to their interests and know they're not alone. For a young person with a strong self-image who's drawn to the positive fetish sites, the Internet can be a great source of support, education and comfort. For the youth with a negative self-image, inclined to seek out the worst, it can, unfortunately, deliver that in spades, from trolls intent on inflicting pain, to women complaining about "pervert" boyfriends.

Community Dialogue:
Do BDSMers still have to hide who they are?

A word about Community Dialogues:

In addition to the in-depth interviews, I wanted to get as broad a perspective on BDSM as possible. For this purpose, I drew on my social media resources. Of my roughly 4,500 Facebook friends, well over half of them are in the BDSM world to one degree or another, from activists and leaders to private players whose only connection to the BDSM world is on the Internet.

In private threads, I asked them to share their thoughts and experiences. Roughly 150+ different people replied across a gamut of ages ranging from early 20s to mid-80s. Participants in the Community Dialogues are identified here only by gender-free initials. I let them speak to their individual experiences of sex and gender identity as they wished, when they found it relevant to do so.

It's a much freer world now, but that doesn't mean that all the myths about BDSM have vanished. Just because more people know about us doesn't mean we have won the war for acceptance. While positive studies continue to stream in, mainstream society still believes what they were told by their elders or their religious leaders. Wide-scale harassment of and discrimination against non-conformist sex and gender expressions remains a norm in conservative communities.

I turned to the Community to find out whether and how discrimination against BDSM/fetish sexuality has affected their daily lives and posed the following question:

Do you feel you have to hide (or separate from daily life) your BDSM/fetish or gender identity?

Respondents fell into three overlapping groups: very hidden, somewhat hidden, and not hidden.

The first group feels compelled to hide their BDSM/fetish sexuality from their employers, their communities or family members for fear of negative repercussions. Some have experienced discrimination in the workplace, while others have had cause to worry about losing custody battles and parental rights.

RG: Yes, because I have to live, work and operate in the "vanilla" world, and they just would not understand.

PA: I was fired once because they discovered my past. I kind of want to stay employed for a little longer.

RWB: Yes, mostly due to employment and child custody concerns. They're more integrated now than they were when my kids were younger, but there's still that worry that I could lose my kids or a way to provide for them if I was completely out.

JD: My ex-husband went on a smear campaign against my sexuality with a folder full of "proof." He presented copies of his evidence that I was immoral and a danger to children to everyone he could. This included my family, my children's friends' parents, the principal of my school, church leaders, the entire Girl Scout council, his attorney, the judge and many more. I had a hard fight to keep custody of my babies. My mother disowned me without any communication with me. My kids' friends found out and made a joke of it. They endured a lot of teasing. I remember walking into a Girl Scout leader meeting and the room got silent. I also fondly remember one mom refusing to look at the evidence folder with the comment, "I lived in NYC all my life. Do you think you can shock me?" It was a painful mess for years. Now I keep it discreet so I can continue teaching.

NED: I live in the Bible Belt. It can be dangerous to be your true self down here. I'm also a Pagan and that part of myself is hidden as well. I grew up in a family where sex was never mentioned. So I learned early on to remain silent about my sexuality.

DR: I keep my gender identity issues to myself and my kinkiness I SELDOM DISCUSS.

WH: I feel based on past experiences that while a small percentage would be interested and an even smaller percentage would be intrigued or curious, the majority of the people I work with or go to church with or my friends would not.

KD: I sometimes hide it. People tend to think I'm doing it for attention and don't realize it's just who I am.

CMM: I definitely feel the need to separate my leather identity from my professional life today, although that wasn't the case in the past. I don't want to lie about it. If someone asks directly, I will disclose, though only if I feel it is safe to do so. I was much happier when I was able to live leather 24/7, and someday in the not too distant future, I know I'll be ready and have the right opportunity to do it again.

A second group tries to integrate BDSM into daily life yet remain deeply aware of the boundaries between public acceptability and private sex/gender choices. They tend to be out within their Communities and with friends or relatives who show acceptance, but still see a need to protect themselves from judgment and discrimination.

JM: There's hiding... and there's just being appropriate. If someone hears a rumor about me and asks, I tell them. No big deal, but I don't get into lurid details, either.

KB: I don't hide but I don't disclose information unless asked. Interestingly enough, most people jump to certain conclusions all on their own, such as that I am a Dom. I usually let them assume whatever they like.

ZLC: I haven't deliberately tried hiding anything since I came out of the kinky closet. I do pay attention to my audience though, simply because I don't want to inflict something on people without consent. I'm pretty sure my job is safe thanks to my union, but I'd rather not test that. People who know me (and know about my kinky bent) know I'm exceedingly dominant. I can't help but have that show through.

SM: While most people in my life know that I'm a collared submissive, they don't understand or respect it. So, with certain exceptions, I tend to keep it as low key as possible around my family. But the clothes or the collar don't make the submissive. It's who I am and it shows, regardless of where I am or who I'm with.

TJE: I think we all have different roles we fulfill in life. When I'm teaching it isn't appropriate for my students to know about my private life, but it would also be a lie to say that I don't use techniques and approaches as a dominant in my classroom and that I don't use my teaching skills as a dominant. Every role I play is a part of me, otherwise I won't accept the role in the first place. I realize that I am lucky in that I can say "no" to roles that I do not feel comfortable with. My slave has to take more of a leadership role in his job than he prefers and it stresses him out so there is more separation for him.

RM: It depends. Do my grandparents know I am a kinky leather chick? No. Do my cousins? Heck, yah!

KK: It really depends on the situation. I recognize how empowering it can be for some individuals to wear their sexual/kink identities on their sleeve. It's just not something I do, except with covert expressions such as wearing leather or meaningful jewelry. Who knows about my identity? My close friend circle, people I attend events with in the kink community and individuals who visit my blog and Facebook pages. Do I tell them all the gory details about my kinks? No, because, for me, that's for my play partner to know and find out. If they need to know, it will come up in our negotiation of the scene. For the most part, other people don't need to know every detail of when or how I fuck my partner.

FM: My policy is not to non-consensually impose information on other people that they haven't asked for. If a person asks me I will answer honestly. This policy leads to a weird mixture of friends and often some humor. If a person becomes a friend they inevitably discover I'm quite kinky. Generally I find it unnecessary to shock the public.

SF: I'm polite and respectful to family and age appropriate to children. I came out to my mother at 19. She was horrified and said, "Please don't mention this again. It will just make me worry. I don't need to know about your sex life." Ever since, we have used the code words "literary club" to mean "Leather club or event." She knows I am an international title holder for "the literary club." LOL. I wear my collar at all times and call my Master "Sir" or "MK" (instead of Master Kevin) in family/vanilla space. I have even had a child come to me and ask me about my collar. I explained that it was, "A symbol of my relationship like a wedding ring." Otherwise, I am happy to have an open, honest age appropriate conversation with anyone who asks, but I do not force the topic on others. I have been outed at work and fired in the past for my sexuality. At present I am very fortunate to work for a large international entity which is very supportive of the LGBTQ people and those of us with alternative sexual orientations.

PM: When I was in a relationship in the past with someone out of state, we didn't need to hide it that much, and could be fairly overt with friends. It was pretty cool. Where I live now, I'm not out about it except with select friends. Even they don't know the complete story. Some people might not be surprised by my sexuality and some family members may have an inkling about it. But people in my circle, even those into "leather," just don't understand my reality. And since it's generally considered shameful for a male, I tend to be very cautious. I don't need any hostility. Humiliation? Not so much.

AL1: Everyone in my life knows that I am a pro Domme and polyamorous. I started stage bottoming when I was 18, and my mom knew – and was concerned but supportive. After literally joining the circus (okay the ren faire) and getting tattoos (and shaving my head...) I knew that nothing I could do would drive us apart – so when I became a pro, I didn't hesitate to tell them. That said, I still do introduce the topic selectively in certain circles – my boyfriends' families know me as a copywriter and production/personal assistant (both of which are also true).

The polyamory is something I don't hide. When I was younger, we tried – but when I accidentally kissed my boyfriend in front of my fiancé's mother, we knew it couldn't continue. Even my grandmother is supportive (I am verrrrrry lucky and come from a secular and awesome family) though she doesn't thoroughly understand.

I use being out as a filtering system – if you can't handle ALL of me, if you don't like me as I am – I don't need you in my life. The exception is the people who I need in my life regardless of their acceptance.

AL2: I adapt things to my audience. For example, my mum knows I am a rigger and I've also spent a while being a rope bottom and she knows I've performed on stages many times, but I call it performance art. What she doesn't know is that during those performances, the person that I tie is usually hurting a lot. Other 'vanilla friends' also know to varying degrees, from 'performance art' through to 'I am a dominant sadist.'

Mostly though, my life is my life. I have no great desire to force my lifestyle choices down anyone else's throats. It's kind of like religion. I respect people's beliefs, and I give them the same courtesy as I enjoy. If anyone asks me questions because they are curious, I am happy to give an explanation.

Sexuality wise, I am openly bisexual and poly. My work knows, my mum knows, everyone knows. That said, I don't work in a position where my sexuality could compromise that. I know many childcare workers (both male and female) who are a part of my local BDSM scene and they would get fired pretty quickly.

A far smaller percent of kinky people are living their BDSM/fetish sexuality in the open. Though they too are mindful of social boundaries and set their own limits on what they say to whom, they integrate their sex/gender identities with their daily lives.

RGH: I don't hide it from anybody (my family knows), but I don't flaunt it to people casually or brag about it either. Especially NOT to younger people under the age of 21. I actually try to avoid vanilla people as much as possible.

AIF: I'm a post-op trans lesbian. I've been out for 20-some odd years. If I wear leather it is my prerogative – fuck them if they don't like it. I still love to top and I occasionally bottom for the right person.

PT: I used to keep quiet about it in my early career, and used a scene name, but I stopped bothering a long time ago (at least 10 years). I'm out to the adult members of my family. Most of my friends are kinky anyway, and the vanilla ones know too. I am a bit cautious about telling new people, but anybody could Google me and find out. On the other hand, I don't have children or work in a kind of job that being known as kinky could jeopardize anything. I can afford to be out.

SS: I'm almost 100% out and thus I need not compartmentalize. I'm blessed to be employed as a corporate attorney and still be out with my employers, who find my BDSM lifestyle interesting and funny (in a loving respectful way). In my vanilla friend circles, I'm mostly out and find, more and more, that they're not all vanilla. In some of my spare time, I serve on the board of directors of a private gun club. I keep a tight lid on my kink in that circle, but not from any fear of being removed from the board. I just don't want the endless practical jokes that would ensue. They'd all be in good fun... these are good non-judgmental people... but I just couldn't handle going into my range bag looking for a holster and pulling out a dildo harness.

NM: I'm one of those weird quirky types, so when someone hears about some new kink, people tend to look in my direction as if that were something I might do or have tried at least once. Usually they're right. On the good side no one is ever shocked and I can have non-judgmental discussions about that kink or some other.

VLR: Luckily, around the time I discovered I was kinky and wanted to identify with the BDSM community, I started my journey towards my doctorate in human sexuality. These paths are tied together for me.

BDT: I came out as gay in the early 80s when that was almost as controversial as kink is today, and I've arranged my life ever since to make sure I'm never trapped in a box. I'm me, take me or leave me. I came out to my mother as kinky when I won my *Drummer Boy* title. I took her out to lunch and slowly circled around to the truth to which she replied, "I kind of thought so. I know gay men are into that." The rest of the conversation turned into an explanation of, "No, Mom, not *all* gay men are into that and a lot of them strongly disapprove." We agreed not to tell my father, because he was rather old fashioned so it would just be one more reason for him to shake his head and say he loved me any way. Later, my mother was so proud of me that she told my father that *Drummer*, a national gay magazine, had given me a regional award for community service and being an outstanding member of my local community. She said he was very proud and got choked up about it.

My brothers found out through mutual gay friends who never considered I might be hiding it, which I wasn't really. My youngest brother's wife is best friends with Ms. Atlanta Eagle 2013 and hangs out at the bar now. We were going out together last week when my nephew surprised me by asking if I minded if he went along, and later rather shocked me when he came out to me by casually asking which gay bar would be good for a first date because he had met a guy he wanted to ask out.

I only have one Facebook page and everybody gets the same Facebook feed. I don't talk about it at work only because details of my sex life isn't work appropriate, although it has come up at one of my jobs and I admitted it.

In summary, it seems that most adults still struggle with how out they can be without negative consequences, while only a handful feel fully free to be themselves.

The only universal in this dialogue about BDSM/gender identity is that most people do not wish to discuss it with or expose it to either children or potentially hostile adults – the former to protect kids, and the latter to protect their own feelings. Indeed, it may be noted at this point that the Community, as a whole, takes a protective view of minors and generally believes that BDSM education should come only after people are old enough to grasp consent issues. Thus it isn't surprising that many of the speakers made note that they avoid revealing their sexual identities to youngsters.

Otherwise, choices about how to live out their BDSM/fetish identity varies from person to person, informed by their personal experiences, where they work, worship, and live, and their individual comfort levels with sexual openness.

ဆ Chapter 2 ဆ
What Really Turns
BDSMers On

You can't talk about sadomasochistic sex without a nod to the origins of the term, and the misconceptions which have sprung from the lasting association between BDSM and the Marquis de Sade. The connection was first forged in 1886 when German psychiatrist Richard von Krafft-Ebing invented the term "masochism," and applied the term "sadomasochism" to describe for forensic purposes the spectrum of people who loved to give and receive pain. It is a whimsically literary term for a psychiatric condition, combining the concept of sadism, i.e. criminal sexual cruelty as depicted by de Sade, with the concept of voluntary male submission as described by 19th century novelist, Sacher von Masoch, in *Venus in Furs*.

While de Sade may be the most infamous person ever to write about power relationships and sexual cruelty, he neither invented the love of pain nor defines it for others. In the ethos of BDSM culture, sadism and masochism are for the mutual enjoyment of consenting adults, while Sadean sex is non-consensual. By conflating consensual SM and Sadean sex, Krafft-Ebing erased the line between consensual sex for pleasure and criminal sex involving a victim. Even today, some forensic psychiatrists view BDSM urges and fetishes as potential indicators of a criminal mentality. This assumption – that all sadism is Sadean, i.e. non-consensual – underlies most of the legal and social prejudice against BDSMers.

A less negative but similarly overbroad bias against BDSM shows up in softer form throughout culture. In today's pop imagery, BDSM is invariably represented by handcuffs and whips. While those toys are, indeed ubiquitous throughout the scene, how people play in private may not include handcuffs, whips or any toys at all. While some private players amass vast and impressive collections of adult toys, they invest in the specific gear that gives them their hottest erotic experience. Simply put, their toys match their fantasies.

The BDSM community comprises an array of specialized sub-communities and within those communities, there is enormous variety in the roles people wish to play, what exactly they enjoy doing, or the type of partner they prefer. Spanking culture is one example. Under the broad category of "the spanking community" there are groups for heterosexuals and groups for homosexuals; groups for people who want romantic role-play with their spanking and for people who only want sensation; groups that focus on male dominance and groups that focus on female dominance and groups for switches, too.

Fetishes account for a good deal of BDSM diversity because fetishes are both ubiquitous and specific. For example, while spanking is a common sex-game, how spankings are delivered (a strop or paddle as opposed to a hand-spanking, standing upright or bent over the knee), can be just as important as the partner one is with, the words used, the roles played, the frequency of play and the clothing worn because arousal itself is an irreducibly subjective experience. No one else can feel turned on in the exact same ways you do. You can only hope that their individual sexual likes and dislikes are compatible with and complement yours.

When we wrote the original *Different Loving*, we let anecdotal evidence drive the organization of material. Our findings in 1991 were that BDSM was a deeply segmented world. Fetishists in particular tended to concentrate on meeting others who shared their specific fetish, rather than, say, leather/D&S culture at large. We organized our book to reflect the small communities which operated, to one degree or another, under the umbrella of "The Scene" yet whose members often had little or no contact outside of their group. Today, it is impossible to segregate the fetishes or organize BDSM according to what people do because BDSM today reflects decades of experimentation and melding of SM, fetish and leather communities.

The consolidation of the sub-communities under the umbrella term "BDSM" gained momentum in the 1980s and 1990s, when activists urged that a united front would make us more effective in preventing unfair police actions and prosecutions that targeted BDSM clubs and practitioners. At the same time, the Internet created unprecedented ease of communication among marginalized fetish communities. As more people entered the Community, BDSM contests and clubs started catering to wider ranges of interests and tastes. Pansexuality – the integration of gay, bisexual, trans, lesbian and heterosexual people in shared BDSM play spaces – began to flourish and further encouraged BDSMers to take a broader view, in general, of what BDSM could be, how many different forms it could take, and how many different ways a body could attain bliss.

Despite intrinsic division along lines of sexual orientation, gender and specific sexual interest, BDSM as a unifying concept, as a political tool, and as the descriptor for a myriad of non-conformist sexual preferences, has been incredibly effective. Unlike the terms SM or sadomasochism, long viewed in mainstream culture as pathological behavior, BDSM is less emotionally-loaded, at once more palatable to the public and more relevant to those who are neither sexual sadists nor masochists. The use of the term BDSM united individuals and groups to seek common cause and friendship across diverse kinks and fetishes.

Another key in the evolution of contemporary BDSM sexuality is that kink culture traditionally encouraged adults to explore their innate turn-ons fully, to experiment with new sensations and fantasies and to use the body as a path to sexual ecstasy and metaphysical states. While sexual variety itself has been demonized in mainstream culture, leading many to opine that opening the door to kink turns into a spiral of depravity, the truth is simpler and more humane. By opening the door to new types of erotic pleasures, adults naturally expand their sexual versatility and discover new sources of sexual and emotional satisfaction.

The extraordinary versatility, complexity, and variety of non-conventional erotic pleasures that are now the entrenched heart of the BDSM experience, i.e. the emphasis on exploring one's physical, psycho-sexual and spiritual potentials through the body, make it impossible for one single label to apply to all. Experienced BDSM players have tried a lot of different things, discovered they like a lot of things, and, in so doing, demonstrated that sexuality continues to shift and evolve throughout our lifetimes, depending upon one's circumstances and opportunities for sexual variety and experimentation.

There is no better way to explore the diversity of BDSM experience than through the real stories of BDSMers.

BDSMers describe their turn-ons

In both in-depth interviews and Community Dialogues, I asked people to talk about the things that turn them on the most. We asked our interviewees, all with over two decades of experience with BDSM, to describe their "personal best" experiences based on long-time experimentations.

Personal bests: 25 years of BDSM

Morgan Lewis HMQ The best story I have was with a submissive. We lived on his yacht for several years. He was so obedient and so submissive to me, yet he was a great lover. We had a great love affair, though we never put it in those words. His submission to me was so automatic, that he knew what to do, and how to do it, to make sure that I was happy. We did a lot of traveling — we sailed from Far Rockaway to Florida on his yacht, and I got to man the boat.

Another very exciting relationship was with a submissive where he was my bride, and we had a whole bridal party and a wedding ceremony. It was the most beautiful thing you could ever see. It was held at Usher's Keep, an SM club that was just opening, and we had our wedding there. One of the bridesmaids was another guy, and one of my friends, who had nothing to do with the scene, but attended the event and fell in love with the maid-of-honor. They are still together today. She wasn't really vanilla, obviously, but the whole event was so hilarious.

I've worked with a lot of cross-dressers. Many of them, you'd never guess. I have all their photos up on my bulletin board and I love looking at their beautiful faces.

Robin Young Oh, goodness. I have had quite a few amazing experiences, but I suppose my top two would be my twenty-seventh birthday, and my tenth wedding anniversary.

On my twenty-seventh birthday, I was at the time in a five-year poly-amorous relationship with one woman, and a five-month polyamorous relationship with another. The two of them conspired to invite five other kinky women of their acquaintance to give me a surprise birthday party. First, my two partners strapped me down to a massage table, mostly naked except for a rubber hood, blindfold, inflatable gag, leather arm sleeves, and leather ankle cuffs. Then they left me there for some time. I could only vaguely hear various noises in the apartment.

Suddenly I felt hands all over me, and female hands at that! They wound up covering me with sushi and fruit, then using me as a lunch table, followed by clothespins, needle play on my cock, and ultimately dressing me girl-style and spanking me until my ass was a solid bruise. Then my two partners enjoyed me more privately later. Absolutely a staggeringly unexpected and completely unforgettable (and almost certainly never to be topped!) day.

On my tenth anniversary, my wife and I spent the weekend at a kinky bed and breakfast in Oregon, and had an incredible time with a glori-ous variety of latex clothing and bondage gear, including some elabo-rate outdoors play – I dearly love playing kinkily outside, but opportuni-ties are extremely hard to come by. Again, an absolutely unforgettable day. I will be less detailed about what exactly we did, but your imagina-tion can fill in the blanks. :-)

Alexis deVille Once, I had one of my submissives role-play as my pimp. It was kind of hilarious. It was a masked ball and I fooled every-one, including people who knew me well. Everyone bought it though, so it was really a lot of fun. I won the contest!

I still have mind-blowing orgasms in my 60s because kink adds so much to the whole. It fills a need in me. It's exciting, still sort of forbidden, even after all these years. Much more exciting to do kink than straight sex.

Nancy Ava Miller I still do enemas on myself all the time, as a hygien-ic procedure. I used to do them professionally as a dominatrix and often educated about it. But these days I just do it for cleansing and health. I consider myself an expert on this. Ironically, when I first got into SM, I was a complete novice at all the different SM activities. So it amazed me when I realized I was already an expert on the enema fetish! That was wild. I seemed to know more about enemas than just about anyone, even the big old leather daddies!

I've played with a lot of different fetishes since then. One of the nicest surprises was when a client asked me for a wrestling session. I was dubious at first. I had never done it, and there was no way I could actually physically overpower him. I kept thinking, "What am I going to do with this guy?!" But it turned out to be such a hoot! He always let me win, of course. He was just really fun and exciting. And physically he was exactly my type: tall, burly bearish kind of man, but not intimidating.

I also had a wonderful client from Georgia, a black guy with very light skin, who asked me to do racial degradation with him. I was really taken aback by that. I couldn't use the N-word with someone! He wanted me to say, "Whip my black nigger ass," and he wanted one of the white girls working for me to fart in his face. And I was like, "Oh nooo, this is too much!" But we nervously started doing the scene he wanted, and he was such a happy, upbeat, playful person, that it ended up being incredibly fun, which I couldn't believe. I can't explain it, but he made it fun by being a truly delightful person.

There was another guy who had a fetish for being frisked. His fantasy was that I'd be a police lady on the street, who stopped and frisked him. Now, when I did prodom, I did 2-hour sessions. So when we did ours, he'd walk back and forth across my bedroom, and I would stop and frisk him. Then he'd walk some more, and I'd frisk him. For two hours. That was all he wanted. Walk and frisk, walk and frisk, on and on it went. I got really bored.

You know, a lot of prodoms say they don't get involved sexually with any of their clients. I don't believe it. If you talk to enough people you find out that a lot of us have allowed a client here or there to lick our pussies. And I love to have my cunt licked.

*Carter Stevens My best hedonistic adventures were my many trips to Europe to shoot videos for my company. I traveled all over Europe, visited many BDSM related clubs and resorts like CLUB DOMA in The Hague. I traveled and enjoyed a first class life of the "Rich and Famous" all while shooting and making money with my videos. It was a hedonistic dream come true.

*Laura Antoniou There's been many wonderful moments of play and connection, some more powerful than others, some with more lasting effects. But to say one or two are favorites? By what standards? I can say that getting my labia pierced at the culmination of a week of intense play was awesome. But so was the first time my hand got into a pussy and the first time it got all the way into an ass. But those are just activities. The first time for anything with my wife matters more than those, even if those moments were transcendent in their own right.

Know what really makes a best moment for me these days? When it's either completely familiar and comfortable and automatic – or it contradicts anything I've done before. Which still occasionally happens.

*Cléo Dubois There have been so many. When energy runs and we merge, both Top and bottom, that does it for me! The air in my dungeon gets electric. We are both 100% present.

One of these peak experiences is actually recorded forever: Right after I ripped the white feathered clothespin zipper off Creed's back in "The Pain Game," we were so focused, the film crew disappeared. As I help her to her feet, our eyes locked. So beautiful and strong in her vulnerability it brought tears to my eyes. In that one I was the caring sadistic Domina. Our love was big. Thirteen years later we are still close!

Fisting: giving and receiving an intimate often misunderstood practice I discovered at the Catacombs a long time ago. Me in the sling, a lover's hand in my cunt surrounded by mainly gay men. I remember cumming, crying, laughing and screaming, "I am home. I am home..." as a "full power bottom."

I have also visited that inner place of deep surrender and belonging in the energy hook pull rituals we do tribally each summer. Pulling on hooks pierced through my skin, topping myself, in community with bright sunshine and the beats of the live drumming. In that trance space I am at core, not top space, not sub space. Words can't describe these ecstatic journeys accurately.

*Lady Elaina I think back to Jim, the man who did the illustrations for my books, who died of brain cancer. We did some incredible scenes together. He liked to do predicament bondage with me. There was a scene with a recliner where I was attached in various places, and he took advantage of me in ways that I could not resist. Move one way and he took advantage of me here, and squirm to get away from that, he took advantage of me there.

Another thing we did was the classic leather wrap-around coat, this time with only a very brief chain harness underneath it. We went out to Paddles [*ed. - New York City BDSM club*], and he attached a leash to the chain that went around my waist and through my crotch, and then hooked the leash over a fence behind where I was sitting. He hooked it a little bit too high, so I ended up squirming to try to get comfortable. You couldn't really see much, but you could see it was attached to something inside that wrap-around coat, but not much more. A crowd of guys gathered directly across from me, clearly hoping to get a glimpse of what was under that coat. Jim deliberately left me sitting there while he went to get us some drinks, taking his sweet time to come back. The rascal. :) It was HOT.

*James My peak DS experience was the entire time of years in service to Ma'am. That was my heaven on Earth. The fact of my service, and the trusting, intimate passion with which She contained me, the way She could receive the gifts of self I brought Her and return them with gifts of Her own Self, is what makes that time stand out for me. My peak SM experiences all took place within the context of that relationship.

One that stands out for me was the hours-long whipping She gave me during which I felt my kundalini rise, when I roared through my pain and roared through my anger and I snapped up and down like a whip or the snake it's named after and ended up floating in a state of bliss I have never forgotten.

*Kiri Kelly If forced to pick, I would say the top two would be both of my collaring ceremonies – because of the events of the evening as well as the emotional significance of giving myself completely.

The first was with the gentleman who I was collared to for a year. The ceremony was held at his friend's home in front of a group of about 35 of his friends and one of mine. I was still new to the local scene so most of the people there were still strangers to me. Everyone there was clothed, but after I was led in wearing a cloak, it was removed and I was naked. After the collaring ceremony, he blindfolded me, tied my hands above me to the rafter and told everyone to enjoy. I was touched, licked, pinched, spanked, flogged, whipped and had all sorts of things done to me... There were times when there were so many hands on me at once that I couldn't tell you how many men or women were touching me. It was also the first time that I had ever experienced electric play and fire play.

Even though I was blindfolded and had strangers doing things to me that I had never felt before, I felt safe. I knew that my Master was watching the entire time and that he knew the expertise level of every-one there and trusted that he wouldn't let anyone cause me any real harm. It was amazing! I had never experienced anything remotely like it before! It was beyond my wildest fantasies and remains today as one of the best experiences of my life.

The other would be the collaring ceremony with my current hus-band/Master, which was an experience on the other side of the spec-trum. It was an intimate evening with just the two of us and was truly the most romantic night of my life. Instead of going down the tradi-tional kinky road as one might expect, he gave me an experience that demonstrated how tender and loving he could be. It was everything that I could have ever dreamed of! We have had some awesome kinky play nights as well, but the tenderness and romance that he displayed the night he collared me touched me to the core.

But if you will indulge me, there is a third experience that also stands out where I had never known such a feeling of wanton exhibitionism. It was at one of the Shadow Lane parties that was held in a ballroom with over 300 people. I was on stage with all of my best friends from the video industry – over the lap of one, with my legs spread and held by two others, my bottom naked and exposed to hundreds of people, while being spanked by Alexis Payne. I can truly say that I didn't want it to end! When she gave me the option of so many strikes with her hand or so many with the crop, I begged for ALL OF THE ABOVE!

slave matt My interest in BDSM from the first has been almost exclusively as a bottom. At first, I was mainly in it for the sensation – the whips, the clamps, etc. It's taken me longer to get into the emotional/subjective aspects of it – the subordination, the pleasure in service. Over the last few years we've gotten into chastity and cuckolding play, which excites me tremendously (though it's unorthodox in that I also have a few outside lovers).

I've found that I can be the same arrogant prick in public that I've always been. It's taken me some time to enjoy teasing and humiliation, since they were sometimes too close to real insults to my ego, but I've been able to separate play from reality much better over the last few years than I used to be. My wife and I have found true love melds well with BDSM. It pervades, though doesn't dominate, our daily life, and it adds so much erotic delight to everything. I realize that I'm very lucky, but there are many ways in which I'm very lucky to have the wife I do. I suppose the challenge is trying to maintain the balance and/or separation between play and reality, but so far so very good. I unleashed my wife's inner sadist, which has been a delight. Best of all is having gone from repressed interest to virtual/fantasy interest, to real life interest. It's so much better this way.

slave feyrie There is no greater high to me in life than reaching a space of total surrender. At first, I found that space in increasingly extreme scenes. Later I found it through slavery so I can LIVE in that space. I exist for that feeling. It is the cosmic ring God put in my nose to lead me around in life. I'm 36 now and will be giving birth for the first time in about a month and a half – and I think this is going to be my most epic moment of surrender and embracing of pain. At least that is my hope. The search of these surrender highs have shaped my entire life.

Community Diaglogue: Turn-ons

A representative example of the BDSM things that turn people on is futile in 2015 because no matter how many you may catalogue, new types of BDSM play, new toys, and new fetishes literally emerge every month – as do new people with new ideas of what's hot. I turned to my Community friends and asked them to list their top five favorites. Results were exquisitely manifold.

What is your top list of BDSM turn-ons?

PR: The stage set (music, lighting, scents). Housekeeping tended (sex sheets, coconut oil in warmer, toys laid out). Full body anointing with warm oil, slow, sensual, lots of cooing, eye-gazing. Moves to toys that scratch, all over my body. When I begin to drop, toys turn to those that thud, take my breath away, drive me deep. Full knowledge that I am safe to drop, my Top will protect me. Long-time breathing, being held, during aftercare.

JM: PR makes a nice point about having the stage set. Nothing nicer than your partner and you putting a bit of work into it.... making sex or play an occasion, and not just something you do because TV is all re-runs. LOL A definite turn on.

BJB: Dressing the part, being in Control, having service offered to Me willingly, being able to inflict pain that brings pleasure, therefore pleasuring Me!!!

JD: 1) cigar play, 2) high protocol (don't ask), 3) rope, always rope, 4) absolute violence, 5) grooming another.

ER: Bondage, caning, Keds, ballet shoes, and Mary Janes.

JK: Watching my wife orgasm, Milking (both male and female versions), latex clothing, shoes, predicament/device bondage.

GG: This is in no particular order: 1. pegging and fisting, 2. interracial sex, 3. man on man rough sex encounters, 4. percussion play, 5. sex positive play parties.

AL: Seamed stockings, lactation, rope bondage, inflatable butt plugs, oral worship.

JW: Body hair and scent.

LM: Okay, these are my unusual ones: being carried like a damsel in distress, having my tears gently wiped away, nursing a man who has been injured in battle or tortured, watching someone get tortured.

KKD: Being controlled/formal protocol, spanking/caning, needles, humiliation/objectification, good aural (listening) sex.

KB: Consensual non consent. Forced or denied orgasms. Breath control. All of those at the same time.

PJD: Tears... not mine, and spanking.

DK: Bondage, blindfolds, face slapping while being taken, flogging/spanking, being taken forcefully.

GS: Aesthetics. Mixes of curves, looks askance, and hair falling just right. Voices. Scent and touch. Silk and satin scarves. Rope. Small whips and slappers. Pleading looks of challenge. Challenging looks of pleading. Sighs. Moans.

MM: Stretching, milking, squirting (male and female), tranny, multiple partners.

SH: 1) Protocol and service, 2) impact play, specifically flogging and caning you, 3) me biting you while kissing you, 4) genital torture, 5) administering golden showers.

AL: Impact play, preferably thuddy (receiving), getting tied up or restrained in some way, hot wax (receiving), sex positive spaces (I'm pansexual and versatile), providing service (these are not in any particular order).

EM: Soft, sensual stimulation ramping up to heavy beating, verbal teasing and pussy spanking. Makes me hot and hard, her wet and whimpering. Yeah, we love the sexy shit.

ACL: Being completely bound with anything soft, silky, furry or latex. Being completely submissive and joyfully willing in group play. Being forced to orgasm to the point of tears. Giving oral to m/f as a form of breath play. Role playing that involves switching to being the Top where I get to plan out a scene makes me especially stimulated for the days leading up to all the surprises (cock/ball torture, cosplay/cross-dressing, breast/vulva torture, spanking, heat play such as electric or wax); I just always do unto others as I anticipate to be eventually done unto me.

BB: Being the object of sadistic anger. Being kicked. Being whipped. Being made to do hard and/or tedious labor. Being burned with cigarettes (all of these acts being done by women).

CH: Service, consensual non-consent, biting/being bitten, handcuffs, gags (especially ballgags)... Yeah, those. *purr*

AL2: Power exchange, breath play, biting, use of brute strength, and the feeling of being found attractive (including hot wife fantasies, etc.).

CMM: 1) Anal sex, 2) Daddy/girl, 3) having a consenting sexual bottom available for me to fuck at my (often) whim.

PB: Male chastity, energy and power exchange, knife play and that wet making feeling you get making someone's body and mind react and then trying to duplicate it. Oh, and gay male fisting porn.

DA: Biting or cutting to blood (then fun things with blood!), service that includes sapiosexytalk, fisting (giving vag & anal, receiving vag). I'm just so predictable.

EH: I'd say *kink zero* is "loss of control," the others are all subsets of it. 1) regression/age play (diapers, crawling, crying, etc.), 2) loss of physical control (diapers again), 3) hypnosis/trance/mind control/obedience/loss of agency, 4) spanking (specifically because it has the effect of pushing me into subspace and/or little space). I was thinking of mentioning consensual non-consent too (the idea of consenting once and then never having the ability to back out of it afterward is a huge button for me) but I guess that's just another flavor of (3) above.

SE: Latex, dressing up, shoes and strap-ons.

TJE: Auctions, service, knives, watching others be sexual upon my orders, and collars.

KPL: Fear, age play, mindfuck, breast play, being of service.

NX: Breath. Constricted, tantalized. Body scent and oils. Water – high consumption to affect duration or breathing, or to warm along with wax or to cool skin and surprise. Intimate sights. Close eye contact, restricted vision. Improvised bondage with scarves, belts, leather scraps, stockings, sheets, tape, string, objects. Controlled suspension.

SW: Service, blood, total control, energy play, boots of any kind on all genders.

AEM: Swords, daggers, scarification (or anything to do with blades and blood) and ROPE!

AL2: 1) PDA especially when he demands in the car on a long stretch of road, on the sailboat under sails, standing in line at amusement parks, at restaurants (he loves long table clothes).... no I'm not just talking about kissing and holding hands. His desire is my command, 2) role-play, 3) being taken (hair pulling, deep throating), 4) whipping/cropping on St. Andrew's Cross or tied to legs of bed, 5) cuddling.

JD: Strict bondage for a longish period of time, hair pulling, when he forces me down to the ground, service, fellatio.

KD: Trying out non-toy items for toy use in public. Not so as to get arrested, but raised eyebrows and whispers get me going. Hearing him mumble to himself while rummaging through the toy bag, not knowing what's coming out next. Being bitten so as to leave marks. Restraints, especially improvised. Consensual non-consent. Role-play.

DEC: A self-proclaimed big bull (BBC) using me solely for his pleasure. Having a Daddy that sometimes throws a bag over my head, cuts my clothes off and then leads me to the playroom where he has set up a gang bang to push me past my limits of endurance, getting fucked so hard and so thoroughly that my legs are like jelly afterwards. Tied to a motorcycle as it barrels down the highway with a big beefy biker fucking the hell out of me (I know it is an impossibility but what can I say

LOL), big beefy cigar smoking Daddy blissfully tormenting my body with his cigar and filling my ass with smoke till I start cramping and then fucking the smoke out of my ass.

CS: My standing line is I love everything about BDSM but I'll give it all up on Thursday for a good blow job. Now for a serious answer... climax control... withholding a slave's permission to climax. Forced climaxes are a real turn on for me.

LH: Gun play, breath play, boots, leather gloves, cigars... and wow, listing only five was a SERIOUS challenge.

RGH: A fist in my hair to focus me, predicament bondage to challenge me, and spanking/flogging/singletail/caning to satiate me.

JGA: Not in any order: nipple play, flogging top and bottom, hanging in jox and smoking cigars, bondage top.

LM: Bondage with flogging (thuddy flogger, of course) and sultry dungeon music. Accompanied by periodic and gentle stroking and snuggling by my Dominant.

JJ: Blood, electrical, fire, and application of intense stimulus to the point of unconsciousness... and all sharp shiny things. Just your average stuff.

KK: Bondage, latex and service (being served).

DK: Smoking, facial hair, good posture, boots, flagging. Although I always smile when people say "whips and chains" because I'm a two-trick pony. I like singletail whips and chain bondage.

Finally, Race Bannon illustrated how incredibly versatile highly experienced BDSMers can become after years of exploring their sexuality without shame.

Race Bannon: Interests (some top only, some versatile, none required): armpits, bears, black, bondage, boys, butt plugs, cam, cbt, chastity (keyholder), chat, cigars, collars, cum, daddies, dark, dildos, dominant, electricity, feet, felching, fisting, flogging, fucking, gang bangs, gear, groups, hairy, kink, kissing, mansmells, masochism, masters, oral, piercing, pigsex, pigs, pimping, piss, public, raunch, sadism, single tails, 666 (fantasy), slaves, slings, sounds, spanking, spit, submissive, sweat, three-way, tit play, torture, vacuum pumping, watersports, wax... and that's the short list.

Sadomasochists on de Sade

Out of curiosity, I also asked the Community about the work of the Marquis de Sade, whose name has contributed so vastly to prejudice against BDSMers. I was curious how many of my 150+ contributing friends thought his work was sexually exciting.

If you've read de Sade, did he turn you on?

PT: I suspect vastly more people have read *about* de Sade than have actually read any of his works.

SJ: I was 14. The book was *The 120 Days of Sodomy.* Thought it had too much shit eating.

RB: I thought I would be shocked in a titillating way and possibly have my "doors of perception" opened. I ended up mostly bored and let down.

JOM: De Sade was an aristocrat who abused women for his kicks, primarily lower class poor women, thus using his aristocratic privilege. The only freedom he believed in was his freedom to abuse lower class women, period.

SS: I was appalled and masturbated in the backseat as my father drove from Santa Fe to Gallup, New Mexico, and my mother read the maps in the front of our car.

PJD: He spoke to me.

KN: Weird dude... but I was quietly tantalized and stimulated. Kinda a hint of things to come for me.

CS: "So much philosophy... this isn't what they said it would be... where's the... OH MY!" Got through *Philosophy in the Bedroom*, *Justine* seemed a little off, but *Juliette* was everything I heard de Sade was supposed to be, with a decent ratio of sex to pages of philosophy, long lists of exotic execution styles and the French equivalent of supervillains engineering famines just because it got them off. Whoa!

FRM: I expected the writing to be better and much longer. I kept thinking, "Is that it?"

DA: I saw it first in snippets in the porn pulp of my early porn reading days decades ago. I thought it "hot" (hey, it was porn), but I really didn't get to read an actual de Sade book until some years later. I read *Justine*, then later, *Juliette*. The scene in *Juliette* I really liked was the description of how the Pope had a sexual circus rigged up in one of the rooms in the Vatican. But, by then I was into the harder stuff myself, so it was more amusingly hot rather than a turn on. Later, when I found out about de Sade's habit of tweaking the noses of his fellow nobles, I started to like the guy.

RS: I find his 'erotic' writings boring. I, like so many others, am captivated by his criticism of rationality.

SF: I liked that he was a fellow pervert. I disliked his actual stories. I'm not into the "treating women like shit then discarding them" genre of porn LOL – I am all about dirty nasty piggy sex scrumptiously seasoned with a dash of humiliation. But truly believing your partner is of less worth as a human being? Nope.

It was the least popular question I asked, drawing the fewest responses. While the mainstream may still misconstrue BDSM as a Sadean world, the reality is that BDSMers are, as a Community, offended by non-consensual sex and violence.

ᛒᴑ Chapter 3 ᴼᴣ
Why Are We BDSMers?

The jury is still out on why some people prefer non-conformist, non-reproductively oriented sex, and particularly acts that seem extreme, such as seeking out intensely painful stimulation or needing to believe in a power hierarchy to be fully aroused. We are still on the frontiers of inquiry into how sexuality is expressed on a biological level.

Certainly, there is a documented history of people doing BDSM and fetish acts going back to early recorded history – body modifications, erotic bondage, fetishism and transgenderism appear in the art of several ancient cultures. In the modern age, the Internet shows that even when we come from completely different backgrounds, environments, families, and classes, there are universal BDSM impulses that bind the most culturally dissimilar people. Internet searches will show that BDSMers in New Zealand are turned on by whips and fetishwear as much as Costa Rican BDSMers and kinky people in Sweden. Is that Internet acculturation? Or is there something intrinsic to BDSM identity that begins at the molecular level?

In research on what role DNA plays in human sexuality and sexual behaviors, a team of epigeneticists led by Dr. Tuck Ngun at the David Geffen Medical School recently announced that they have developed an algorithm with a 70% accuracy rate in predicting whether a man will be gay or straight based on a molecular marker. Whether this algorithm will hold up under further testing is unknown as of this writing, but the possibility that DNA plays a role in adult sexual identity is gaining traction. BDSM scholars certainly are wondering if future science will reveal genetic markers for kinks, masochism, fetishes, and other seemingly innate preferences.

Brain scientists meanwhile are studying neural pathways for data about sexual behaviors. A 2015 brain imaging study at Rutgers University suggested, according to study author Barry Komisaruk, that there is "a fundamental link between pain and orgasm pathways." Scientists are calling this connection "benign masochism." It means that the human brain perceives some painful experiences as both innately desirable and fundamentally harmless and consciously engages in seemingly painful experiences. Benign masochism only appears in humans – other species apparently don't choose to eat chilies that burn their mouths, walk on fire, or take spankings. Still, exactly how it applies to BDSM has not yet been studied, though the link is scintillatingly suggestive.

Ironically, the idea of an innate BDSM identity was first floated by 19th century Krafft-Ebing, who suspected there was some underlying biological explanation for the population of people with sexual perversions. He concluded that people were likely born with a perverted constitution, and then influenced by their nurturing and traumatic life experiences. If we remove the negative assumption that all non-conformist sex is perverse, and the unfounded belief that trauma is a necessary component of growing up kinky, the theory still holds some water.

In my book *Sex for Grown-Ups*, I made the case that BDSM/fetish sex should be viewed as a class of sexual identity, with characteristics common to all. I based it in part on the new medical research, as we now know that the brain is filled with differentials that enable different capacities, responses and sensitivities in different people, creating true individuals.

At the same time, DNA is not a prescription for life: human experience shapes sexuality too. Many people see their path into BDSM/fetish as a journey into pleasure and/or pain, much as mountain climbers looking for their next hellish peak or cheese lovers seeking out the most wretchedly redolent gorgonzola money can buy. The journey itself, though, is different for each person. Mistakes, accidents, wrongful assumptions, trauma, and anxiety can alter the course of an individual's sexual journey, just as affirmation, positive re-enforcement, pleasure and orgasm will also shape a person's sexual turn-ons.

Since data on whether BDSM is genetically encoded, a function of the brain, and how much is nature v. nurture v. evolving adult sexuality are both sparse and unreliable for now, anecdotal evidence is still our best source of realistic perspectives on how and why people get into BDSM.

I asked our in-depth interviewees,

How did you first find your way to BDSM?

*James I have been interested in the BDSM lifestyle since I was old enough to think about sex. I can't imagine I ever looked seriously at relationships through any other lens. So you might as well ask: How has being male impacted me? How has being white impacted me? How has being an oxygen breathing mammal impacted me? This is how and who I am, and it is how I understand relationships in general.

*Constance-Marie Slater When I started out, I knew nothing. I had only discovered that it was inside me. As I wrote in my book, *Kaleidoscope*, I was surprised when a male friend said, "You're such a bitch, you should be a dominatrix." And I said, "I would never hurt anyone." And he said, "Hurting is not necessarily harming." So I went and I learned, and I discovered that I am a switch.

*Carter Stevens I was a "professional pervert" (i.e. a pornographer) when I first started to dabble in BDSM. It didn't affect my private life a whole lot until I started publishing the *S&M NEWS* monthly national newspaper in the late 80s. Then my private BDSM life took off like a rocket. I started making appearances on TV shows like Sally Jesse Raphael and Phil Donahue billed as a BDSM "expert" and suddenly submissive females were seeking me out. With all this practical experience and lots of reading on the subject I did acquire a certain amount of knowledge. I also started starring in many male Dom BDSM videos for companies like Gotham Gold which only added to my stature as an "expert" male Dom.

*Cléo Dubois Rather than remaining victimized by the intensely negative programming and abuse I suffered in my childhood and teens, I escaped. I came to San Francisco, not knowing what I would find. SM sex and freedom found me. In 1982 a devoted lover who suspected I was kinky escorted me to Kat Sunlove's ground breaking class on female dominance. In that small San Francisco anarchist bookstore, I discovered a part of me that was ready to come out. Kat recommended the Society of Janus as the portal into my new world. I joined eagerly, attended every meeting and, volunteering as a demo bottom, I got to feel what it was like. Quickly my explorations took me to both sides of the whip.

Home among Leatherfolk at the Catacombs (I'm Carla in the book *Leatherfolk* by Mark Thompson), I found my fire, my voice and my heart. Informed consent was the key that opened the door to my reclaiming, healing and personal power.

Stephanie Locke I knew as a child, even from my earliest memories, that I was fated to be dominant over men. My mother inspired men – extremely beautiful and tall, well educated, she looked like Ingrid Bergman and dressed exquisitely too. I remember being about three when a man approached my mother on the bus and began complimenting her feet. I was amazed but my mother, ever the lady simply said, "Thank you." I remember I looked at my little feet in blue jellies, and they looked exactly like my mother's feet. This meant I had beautiful feet too. And suddenly I realized that anything could be pretty to a man. That understanding – that it didn't have to be your hair or face, that every part of a woman was beautiful – really sank in and stuck with me. I knew there would always be ways for me to be beautiful to men.

I had an active imagination. When I was around nine, digging around my parents' home, I found my way to some old-fashioned magazines and novels with, what I later realized, were very kinky plot lines. They fascinated me. I read one story that described a posh secret club in

New York, attended by a Mistress who had slaves who waited on her hand and foot. I read that story over and over. This was what I wanted for myself! When I grew up, I wanted to be a woman like that, a woman who had slaves. I started dreaming and plotting how to become one of the greatest Mistresses in the world.

Lolita Wolf I started out by calling phone sex lines in the latter part of the 80s, and got warned away from the organized scene. People said don't go to TES, so I started going to clubs – the Vault and Paddles. It wasn't organized but I started going every weekend. Then I tried going to TES once, when they were meeting in a strip club. There was only me and one other woman and it was really creepy. And this guy got up and started telling his own story about how a Mistress wouldn't listen to him, and she ended up breaking his collar bone. This was my first time so I thought "no way" and I left. Then I was at a club about a year later, and I met Hilton who had a TES table. He invited me and I went back: this time it was a nice clean space above the strip club, and there were other women, so it was much better.

I did a lot of flip-flopping around back then. I didn't know anything. I started out on the bottom side, and met someone who I bottomed to, and he taught me how to top. Then I found more people to teach me things, and I became more of a top. I was really a switch: in those days, people thought you weren't "real" if you identified that way. So I became a "top who occasionally rolls over." It took me a while to finally say I am a switch, but it was hard because I was going against the stream.

slave feyrie I had a lot of fantasies in my childhood which I expressed in games, fantasies and drawings. But I did not have my first "scene" until I was 13 years old – with a boy my same age who had similar fantasies which we had confided in each other. I did not understand or know that there were words or labels for what we did until I got onto AOL. Then I lied about my age and called myself "girlsub27" to get people to talk to me.

When I was 16, a boy 2 years older than I, with whom I had an online "relationship" was becoming active in the BDSM community. He made me aware that there were "groups" out there for people like me. Meanwhile, though I was mainly attracted to the submissive role, I started exploring my top side and began "enslaving" boys in my high school and the occasional girl.

slave matt My first perverse stirrings were in front of the Stations of the Cross in my hometown Catholic church. The Stations are a feature of most Catholic churches that depict the crucifixion of Jesus in great detail, including the crown of thorns he was made to wear, the whipping, the public humiliation, his being nailed to the cross and stabbed in the ribs. Lots of glorious suffering, yes, but combined with the grandiosity of being the Son of God and the Savior of Humanity – a combination known and loved by bottoms everywhere. I was only about 12 at the time and while I knew that I was excited, I didn't really understand why and didn't think about it for years.

I started figuring out what those strange stirrings were all about when I got to college and discovered the Velvet Underground and their song "Venus in Furs" ("kiss the boot of shiny shiny leather/whiplash girlchild in the dark"). From that I went on to read *The Story of O.* So I developed a name for and understanding of my outlandish desires but never acted on them for years afterwards.

Deborah Addington I had my first kinky experience when I was around 5. I got the kids I was playing with to carry me around on a chaise lounge and fan me with palm fronds because I was Cleopatra. My playmates did not enjoy this game as much as I did; I didn't really understand the principles of consent at that age. By the time I was 17, I was fully engaged in BDSM with partners, experimenting wildly and using whatever was at hand. My first exposure to organized BDSM was in the early 90s in San Francisco. I went into A Different Light bookstore and found a copy of *SM 101* by Jay Wiseman, when it was a homemade-looking, spiral bound 8.5"x11" book. I realized that book being published at all was proof that there were other people like me out there, who liked the same sex things I did and were thinking deeply, exploring safely. I fully realized that I was not alone.

Nigel Cross I was probably in my late teens when I first started to realize that normal relationships were never going to work for me. One of my earlier girlfriends, who was far more knowledgeable about such things than I ever could have been, recognized that much of our interactions involved how I could best do things for her, quite often at a loss for my own needs. She took to calling me her "submissive" even though we never really took it any deeper than that. Had we remained together in the years to come, I'm sure it would have developed that way.

My first BDSM relationship occurred while I was attending the United States Military Academy at West Point. My squad leader was a woman who immediately recognized that I was a submissive. Whenever my squad leader and I were alone, she often chose to have me take a position of attention on my knees before her, rather than just standing, which was definitely a departure from standard procedures at the Academy. At one point she told me she recognized me as a submissive, and that if we were in any other context, she would have collared me as her slave.

Guy deBrownsville Though I had first learned about elements of kink in the mid 1980's, I didn't pursue it or identify as kinky until much later, in the late 1990's. Someone I was dating introduced me to the *Sleeping Beauty* trilogy by Anne Rice and took me to a few clubs. When our relationship fell apart I found a couple of other people who were kinky, but we were not a part of any community or lifestyle. After being a 9/11 first responder, I took a different outlook on life and when I saw an ad on the back page of the *Village Voice* for the Eulenspiegel Society (TES), an ad I'd mulled over for years, I finally decided to take the plunge and go. I joined my first night. I think that was in 2004.

Chrissy B. I was irresistibly drawn, at age 13, to peep shows – which were really tame by modern standards – and then, when men wanted to fool around with me, agreed, but asked them if they had any lingerie for me to wear. I didn't really know the label "kinky" for some time thereafter, and now I probably wouldn't regard it as "kink" per se (that would have been a couple of years later, when restraints and "forced" femme fantasies emerged). Or perhaps I got my first inkling of what was to come by exploding into a spontaneous orgasm the second time I slipped on a pair of panties at age 8. Don't have a clue why I put them on. But I did, and the rest just followed.

Karen Kalinowski I think I have always been kinky. I remember enjoying the sensation of sticking needles through the tips of my fingers from age 10. Also, I distinctly remember playing Mistress-slave games with a boy a couple years my junior as a child. The theme varied (i.e. Sinbad scenes taken from comic books, etc.) but I was always in the situation where he was in service to my requests. I do believe that sexual abuse, which occurred to me at an early age (between ages 3-8), colored the way I currently play and how I positively reclaimed my sexuality. Being able to control aspects of play (even when I sub for my partner) is still relatively important even though my trust in him is absolute.

Justin Tanis I began exploring BDSM as a college student in New England and discovered leather shops and books in Boston in the mid-1980s; I was aware that there were leather bars but didn't visit them. However, my personal experiences of BDSM were limited to a network of friends and friends of friends, and not connected with any public gatherings, so I wasn't a member of any organizations until I moved to San Francisco in 1994. At that point, I became involved in the Journeyman II Academy and participated in the San Francisco leather community, and then in the communities in Los Angeles, Washington, D.C., and back to San Francisco. (If there were leather spaces open to women in Massachusetts and Hawaii, the places I lived in the late 80s/early 90s, I wasn't aware of them.)

When I was first able to do a BDSM scene with another person at 19 (my fantasies and daydreams started much earlier in adolescence), I wouldn't say that I had an identity related to BDSM, only a desire to experience different sensations and activities. This was mainly, but not exclusively, as a bottom, although I didn't know that word for the first couple of years. I mostly wanted to see what my body could feel, do, learn and revel in. In Brazil a few years ago, I bought a magnet that said in Portuguese, "the body is a celebration." That definitely expressed how I felt and feel.

We then turned to the Community for their insights about BDSM identity and whether they think it is an ingrained orientation or a learned behavior.

Do you think you were "hard-wired" for BDSM?

GRF: From over 2,000 responses to my own Fetish research survey, about 65% stated they were "born this way," about 29% felt it was from their environment.

UA: I believe I was hard-wired. I started having (wonderful) power dynamic fantasies starting at age 11 (perhaps 10) not being attributed to a life event (watching or getting a spanking, etc.). Certainly it was enriched after I ran across soft core porn (*Argosy* magazine, etc.), then increasingly harder core porn. Then I got into the physical aspects and realization of it – finally joining the Community in 1980, and have been in it since. Still there were so many life distractions that could have deviated from my lifestyle, but I always stuck with it. That to me is hard wiring. The same for my being at heart a Master.

TW: Yeah, me too. I don't remember anything that really triggered it, my parents were straightforward and honest about sex, I was never abused or anything else people say are the cause of being kinky. I just am.

DDK: No idea. Happy childhood, loving parents and grandparents. I was doing self-bondage before age ten and I can probably give you a fairly complete catalog of BDSM-oriented storylines and scenarios in Saturday morning cartoons.

PA: I grew up on a farm in Montana. I had no outside BDSM influence and yet from a very young age I drew pictures of women tied up and used to practice self-bondage. But I never saw any images or read any writings until I went to school in Arizona, where I came across pictures and writings and met a girl who was already kinky, not one who I had introduced to kink. When I moved out here to Seattle, it was the first time I saw latex in real life, and the first time I found stores where I could purchase bondage gear. It was amazing to see in real life what I had fantasized about and thought up and created myself much earlier.

DR: I do think there are elements which predispose me to certain forms of BDSM. And from communicating with other kink-identified people, I think that's generally true. That being said, I think "hard-wired" is a somewhat simplistic metaphor, even for gender-based attraction (gay/lesbian, bisexual, hetero). I tend to think of an individual's sexuality and/or sexual orientation as a symphony, with biological and other innate factors serving as the "score," and our more conscious actions as more subtle "arrangements" and "performances."

JM2: In my case, I think it was the simplicity of it that was the main attraction: as an adolescent, I found sex to be really complicated. Then I came across this photo spread on the movie of *Story of O* in one of my father's *Playboy* magazines, and I was immediately struck by how well defined things were: the roles, the expected behaviors, the reward/punishment dynamic. It seemed not just "right," but obvious! When I finally had a chance to try it, I suddenly felt like my sex life was firing on all cylinders. I'm not sure if I am "hard-wired" for it, but to me at least, it was like riding a motorcycle after spending a lifetime walking in a desert. Why go back to something (like mainstream sex) when it's so... unsatisfactory? Oh, and by the way, I'm a submissive.

PM: A minor incident with other kids when I was about 4 indicated I might be hard-wired. As a slightly older kid I was transfixed by various things in media like "Emma Peel" of *The Avengers* in action in a leather "cat suit" etc. As an older teen I discovered evidence that my father was an enthusiast, different role, different orientation. Whoa! WTF? Genetic?

SF: I am hard-wired this way – was playing sexual SM games with myself and fantasizing – including drawing pictures from age 3. I am pretty sure I still have childhood drawings of SM fantasies at my mother's house – and the only imagery I was exposed to even remotely related were crucifixion images at Sunday school – and why would I react like I did vs. how most other children reacted? Wiring methinks.

RB: I'm hard-wired. I need pain to achieve orgasm and am turned on by pain. I've had that reaction ever since I can remember experimenting with my own body as an adolescent and it's been a part of every intimate relationship I've had. I view it as much a part of my sexual orientation as being bisexual. Power exchange I think is more of a proclivity for me. I'm attracted to power imbalances and thrive in relationships that promote them.

BB: For me I think it was hard-wired. Just a random alignment of neurons due to a random array of DNA. Having said that... I love to tell this story: I was once killing time (procrastinating) in the NYU Bobst Library decades ago. I decided to look through some old psychoanalytic literature to see what those types had to say about the origins of sexual sadists, masochists, and fetishists. I found a paper from the 50s in which the writer had a theory, based on her male patients with fetishes, to explain fetishism in men. The theory was quite convoluted. But the common thread was that her male patients with fetishes all had an amputation or similarly bloody accident at a certain age. (A symbolic castration, the theory goes.) Anyway it was a bit of a eureka moment as I, a fetishist to no small degree, had such an accident. The tip of my pinky was cut off by a door at age 3 or so. Despite certain flaws in her theory and questions about psychoanalytic theory in general, I did have to say hmmm to this.

JM: I was absolutely hard-wired this way. I can't remember a time I didn't fantasize (and act on those fantasies) about all sorts of things – and I'm talking as a 5-year-old.

KB: I'm not sure why I'm into the s/m part so I do believe I'm a hard-wired masochist. However as to the D/s part of me? Also hard-wired because being a slave is by no means easy but it's so fulfilling to me. I think perhaps because I so desperately wanted to make everyone happy. I still do but it's much more tempered with the knowledge that some people will only be happy when they're miserable and have something to complain about. However, I am still on the search for the One who deserves me and my desire to be a slave.

GW: I have no clue as to *why* I am a sadist. I just know that the earliest sexual fantasies I can remember involved kidnapping women and torturing them. Fortunately, I wanted to stay out of prison badly enough to not actually do any of that sort of stuff until found someone who liked the idea of having that sort of thing done. And until I got very clear consent to do so.

ER: Television experiences with 1950s TV shows such as *Terry and the Pirates* which included "The Dragon Lady" and *Sky King* which included Penny who was tied up every week. Also several experiences with bondage from a lovely female cousin a year older than I all contributed. Cowboys and Indians games in which astonishingly I seemed to always be the one tied to the tree sealed my fate I guess.

WH: Even before puberty I loved to play spanking games. My earliest masturbatory fantasies involved spanking. I can enjoy sex by itself but it is better with spanking as foreplay. I tried therapy and sex addiction support groups, and took a 7-year break from spanking, but my desires were too strong.

RG: I grew into it with exposure to the gay community through my partner and his friends (I've always been a loner). I can play Dom (preferred) or sub, but I refuse to be bound or tied up; I similarly have an issue giving up that much control to anyone but my (ironically, uber-vanilla) partner, who would NEVER have any interest doing fun things like that.

DF: I knew I liked certain things a whole lot more than I should at a very young age... long before I knew I liked women... I may not have had the vocabulary to explain it to anyone as a kid... but, looking back, it was obvious I was a little perv.

TJE: BDSM fit into a world view I developed when I was a child for a variety of reasons. But unlike standard hierarchical relationships, BDSM had a central theory of mutual consent and choice that was lacking in most justifications for hierarchies. Basically, it felt natural for me to be in a dominant role even though I was raised in a patriarchal society and in an abusive family, and BDSM gave me permission to feel good about those feelings.

RGH: At age 8, my dad told me he really wanted me to be a boy. From that day on, I could never "please the daddy" (straight A student, goody-goody, always trying), but no matter what I did, our relationship was anything but a good one. Haven't talked to him since I was 22. I think being given the opportunity to finally allow my submissiveness to come out actually saved my life, in all honesty. I am very happy to have a husband (Dom) that understands that about me, too.

CMM: BDSM is a spiritual path for me, and one that I happened upon at age 18; although I do believe I would have found my way to it eventually, regardless. I readily acknowledge that I'm a minority in BDSM, being that it is not a primarily sexual experience for me. I do think I'm hard-wired for some aspects of BDSM, specifically masochism, sadism, sexual topping, and service; dominance and submission have always been roles that are primarily in response to the energy of another for me (in the context of BDSM, as opposed to the Butch/Femme dynamic). Who and what I am is complicated, and yes, hard-wired.

FM: I tend to believe that a person's first sexual experience creates their sexual template. Under the age of two my mother had me in the top drawer of a short dresser as a makeshift crib. There was an earthquake and the dresser fell onto me. They put me in a torso cast and the doctor whimsically fashioned a plaster handle to my back. This means I was carried around face down and 'people' had access to my genitals (changing diapers). Later, as a girl under the age of two my parents commonly allowed visiting adults to hold me. One, in particular, liked to diddle under the dress. I've had lifelong interest in consent issues and have progressively sought total control in access to my body. Please note that a sexual experience doesn't need to be sexual (such as changing diapers) – as a tiny child I had no concept or context for sexuality – but, it was how I was touched and necessarily I'm certain it felt good to be changed. Pleasure, restraint and consent problems morphed into my adult self. I tried being submissive for a very short time until I realized my husband had no clue what my experience was (making me feel unsafe) – so I switched to topping.

KK: Hard-wired for certain but then again I wonder if it's a matter of perception. What is "normal" for children? Who defines what is kink and what is vanilla? How many kids play doctor (medical exploration fantasy), cops and robbers (bondage), rough housing/grappling and even rape play? I remember all of that as being "games" that were played. Reading a Sinbad comic also led to some very exotic play scenes that you wouldn't typically think as children's play.

JD: I'm definitely hard-wired, but "nurture" also encouraged my submissive nature.

ZLC: I'm definitely hard-wired. According to my mom, I've always been bitey (still love it). I remember this one time when I was about 4-5 and my (same age) cousin had pissed me off, so I grabbed a cattail from the ditch and chased him and hit him on the backs of the thighs and cackled wildly as he ran screaming, "Hey, stop! That hurts! Stop it!" I've also always been drawn to the leather lifestyle though didn't realize it was mainly because I fall under the trans umbrella and LOVE bears. At 13+, I was drawing very kinky scenes with leather-clad gay men including incest (twins), threesomes, gangbangs, and bestiality. Had my teachers seen that, I'm sure I'd have been sent for massive amounts of therapy.

RT: I was always a sexual child. At 5 my parents had to inform me to go to my room to do what was effectively masturbating... I believe I was always drawn to the scene because, I think, smart creative people have better sex lives due to more active imaginations that contribute to fantasy and reality. I always enjoyed porn and erotica. I believe I personally was drawn to being a sub solely based on my first sexual experience. I was very inexperienced in practice, but not in words. He took me from behind and I had no idea we were having sex until I realized both hands were on my shoulders. Somehow that experience translated into being turned on by dominance.

ACL: I was born with hormones on steroids. I started slow at the age of two with self-stimulation to go to sleep. My older sister would get pissed and call for my mother to make me stop. At three I started exploring gender roles with my same age girlfriend. We played boyfriend/girlfriend and took turns with the roles. By four I became fascinated with an older boy and I asked him to let me suck his "thing" the way I sucked my thumb; he accepted and that led to further exploration and play. I continued to develop rapidly and started trying different ways to satisfy an ever growing hunger by using everyday objects (prickly hair rollers, a fur coat, Bobby pins, spoons, clothespins and the door knobs were no longer safe). I got my period at nine and then became insatiable. I was living a very normal well-adjusted childhood with a secret twist. I started playing with restraints, mentally and physically with leather belts and men's ties. I would make up games where I became restrained. It was a relief to not be responsible for my appetite. Then at twelve I talked my female friend and her brother's best friend into a three way and I suddenly found where I fit. I had an innate need to have multi-dimensional relationships and power exchanges. I married a twenty-eight-year-old when I was eighteen and he allowed me the maturity of a safe, sane and consensual D/s relationship. I am now fifty and in my third marriage of 11 years. Before we married, my husband agreed that I could keep my BDSM poly relationship with another married couple as long as I was happy. So now I have the world with two separate multi-dimensional relationships built on mutual respect. I'm still exploring.

JK: At age 5 I remember having my first BDSM related dream, predicament bondage... spider webs, deep mud and a girl from kindergarten were all part of it. From then on I would practice self-bondage and stimulation, including anal. I really think I'm wired for it

RM: For me it is all about trust and how utterly erotic I find it when I trust a Domme. In "everyday life"... I trust nobody. I don't think I am hard-wired this way as I was introduced to the scene at the age of 40 on a night out and have never looked back, but before that night I had never thought or fantasized about being submissive in any shape or form.

BF: I know I was into being restrained, and excited by fantasies of torture and domination, for as far back as I can remember. Sometime around age 6 or 7 I persuaded my sisters to tie me up and pull down my pants – which they couldn't see the point of because we dressed and bathed together all the time, but it excited me fiercely. On the other hand, I don't believe in genetics here. One of the things that makes humans so adaptable is that we have to learn a lot of things other species know by instinct, and I think one of those things is how to have sex. And it's probably butterfly-wing random influences at the earliest age that determine whether we end up on the middle of the bell curve of normal or out on the fringes.

Clearly, BDSMers often trace the roots of their interests to childhood, reporting that they were always inclined to gravitate towards non-conventional sex. Until the science catches up with us and can deliver circumstantiated data on the biology of sexual diversity, it's fair to say that the anecdotal evidence shows that most BDSMers believe they were born to be sexually different.

∞ Chapter 4 ∞
Real BDSM Lives

Since sadism and masochism first came to the attention of 19th century psychiatry, there has been an unchecked assumption that BDSM/fetish lives and relationships are fraught with instability and dysfunction. This is the result of unfounded psychiatric assertions that all kinky people are mentally ill and that, being mentally ill, they will be not be able to lead stable, healthy lives, much less to build mutually-rewarding relationships. The toxic myth that BDSM relationships are doomed to fail has poisoned many people against embracing their authentic needs for BDSM and fetish sex.

In a very intriguing 2015 study, Czechoslovakian researchers surveyed 192 urban European adults to find out, *"Why do some women prefer submissive men?" (Jozifkova, Konvicka, Flegr J, via the National Center for Biotechnology Information)*. The researchers concluded that a dominant/submissive dynamic in a couple – regardless of which gender was dominant – improves a married couple's long-term cohesiveness and reproductive success. Researchers speculate that a dom/sub dynamic in a marriage makes sex more arousing and that further study could yield data on the evolutionary biology of sadomasochism.

Our anecdotal research backs the research data: we found that there is tremendous stability, loyalty and kinship among kinky people, and remarkably few divorces or breakups among long-time partners. Even among couples who separated, the love and emotional commitment seldom dies.

In "The Leather Menace" from 1982, cultural anthropologist and leather scholar Gayle Rubin first articulated the idea that "Leather is thicker than blood." This sentiment that has since been echoed by many leather activists. It speaks to the sense that being BDSM is an identity that brings with it certain understandings, a certain kind of loving compassion for your partners, perhaps even a special kind of altruistic bond to other BDSMers. When you add the sexual dimension – that BDSMers seek out nakedness and vulnerability without inhibition in their intimacy – the overall sense that we are bound to together plays out powerfully not only in our organizations and clubs, but in our personal relationships and commitments to one another.

For those who are not entrenched in the BDSM world, and for newcomers easily blinded by all the shiny toys, the biggest obstacles in forming solid BDSM relationships are that first, there are few if any role models for how kinky relationships work. We are surrounded with advice on how to make vanilla relationships work but when it comes to building a relationship with a fixed power dynamic or unusual sexual practices, most BDSMers recognize that they will have to create their own models.

There are some advantages to this. Perhaps the single greatest benefit is that it compels people to negotiate, communicate, and forge workable compromises from myriads of small details, such as the language they use in private versus public, to who does which household chores, to the toys they will incorporate into their sex lives. By articulating all their personal desires and requirements, most BDSMers overall end up having healthier relationships than traditionally married people, who may never communicate deeply about their true needs. The risk is when those conversations do not take place. Lack of clear and fully mutual communication makes truly informed consent impossible.

A second obstacle to BDSM relationships is that many newcomers base their ideas of what BDSM is (or should be) on erotic novels, porn websites, and professional domination sites. The fantasies woven tend to portray lifestyle slaves/submissives as being one-dimensional "gimps," a la *Pulp Fiction*. It would be an amusing conceit if it was not so widely perceived as real life. While there are Community groups which document and disseminate accurate leather history, most notably the Leather Archives and Museum (a Chicago-based collection of documents and artifacts), the Internet remains awash in fabulists who concoct false histories and self-appointed gurus seeking converts by claiming to hold the gospel on what BDSM is or should be. Recent books, movies and media representations of BDSM have only added to the confusion about consensual, loving kink by frequently conflating BDSM and interpersonal violence.

There is now increasing attention to and discussion within the Community about the need for more education on the warmth and humanitarian relationships that spring from BDSM. As the interviews show, one of the hallmarks of a successful BDSM relationship is flexibility and openness to change, both in roles and how those roles are defined.

We're also seeing more and more adults willing to share information about the realities of life as a BDSMer, from dealing with children and parents to dealing with arguments or jealousies that may arise. Certainly there is a greater understanding, especially in younger generations of kinky people, that the old rules – or what people once considered to be the rules – no longer apply, and that BDSM is more about creating an original template for one's sexuality than stepping into a pre-ordained pigeonhole.

Being in a BDSM relationship, or even a Master/slave relationship, does not mean following unrealistic ideals, or trying to conform to any one Community standard. It is a more anarchistic, nuanced and intimacy-based construct which allows people to be their best selves, according to the dynamic that makes them feel the most at peace. Whether that is the gay Master/slave relationship that follows strict Leather protocols or the androgynous poly/fetish couple who switch roles on a whim, it's about finding the right partner and creating your own definition of joy. Put another way, BDSM is not about doing BDSM according to someone else's rules: it's about people harnessing their kinks to create their personal vision of happiness.

To understand the realities of life as BDSMers, you have to hear from people who live it. We asked all 31 of our in-depth interviewees to tell us about their personal journeys in kink. We carefully selected our interviewees, limiting them to reliable sources whose personal and relationship histories we know can be verified. Nineteen of them are people who participated in the original *Different Loving* (indicated by an asterisk before their names). All of them have been self-identified BDSMers for 20 or more years. They are arranged in age groups, from oldest to youngest, with our most senior contributor currently age 85 and our youngest contributor age 37. Our pansexual mix of interviewees are an ethnically diverse sample of heterosexual, bisexual, gay, lesbian, trans, and polyamorous BDSMers.

Together, they provide an historical perspective on the realities of BDSM lives. They show that while there is no single gospel, no "right way to do it," and no magic formula, there is a powerful potential for incredible personal happiness in BDSM.

BDSMers 80+

*Fakir Musafar

At age 85, Fakir is both the oldest and most experienced of all our interviewees. He is a pioneer of radical sexuality and the father of Modern Primitivism.

My transformation to Fakir began with severe physical experiences that began at age 12. I was called Roland back then, and was totally isolated but had stories and pictures and movies to inspire me. My question as a kid was, "If other people did this, why did they do it?" Roland had an empathic connection with people in the pictures, and a growing sense that western ideas about the body were bullshit. So he secretly began to use his body just to see what would happen.

The biggest lesson of my own journey is that your body belongs to you: it doesn't belong to God or your mother. The premise that your body doesn't belong to you is very Christian. A modern primitive is someone who said bullshit on that old religious ethos. We say, "This is my body, I have a right to do with it as I wish." The only exception is if it would interfere with someone else's life.

My message as an adult is that you can shift your consciousness through a radical physical experience. Don't say no to anything. Try everything that appeals to you. Your body belongs to you and only you because you're the person inside. And for Christ's sake, learn about what the people before you have done. Respect the elders who have lessons to teach.

People today recognize me as a pioneer in several areas. For example, I'm considered a pioneer in corseting because, in 1959-1961, I began working on a revival of corseting. That revival took hold, and social media has been a huge factor in creating the shifts. I'm in a tight-lacing society which started on Facebook with 30 members, and which now has thousands of members because of the power of the Internet. Another area where I'm considered a pioneer is bondage suspensions: there are now hundreds of groups and people are doing this on a daily basis. I was an early pioneer of body modifications and body play. We founded "Fakir's Intensive Body Piercing School" in 1991 to meet the growing interest, and now we have students on standby because we can't offer enough classes to meet the demand. It's become an institution in that world, not a personal project, which is how it began.

One of the difficult parts of being a pioneer is seeing things get perverted. Many of the big conventions have turned into big fetish shows. A lot of us who attended events even 10 or 20 years ago might not recognize any of the new people. Frankly, people are doing modifications today that scare the hell out of me. So sometimes they take things to new extremes that may not be good for them in life, like earlobes stretched down to people's shoulders. Body modification is filled with layers and depths most people don't understand. All of these practices have much deeper spiritual sides. But we live in a culture today where everyone thinks everything can be done instantly – and that it's all reversible. It isn't. Still, I also see many improvements: improved quality of tattoos and body piercings, and a much higher quality of piercing jewelry – you can find beautiful ornaments in real gold and silver now.

I celebrated my 85th birthday in 2015. I have a wonderfully close and loving partnership with my wife, Cleo. The older we get, the more gentle we learn to be with each other, and the more we honor our bond. If I was talking to Fakir circa 1991, I'd tell him not to feel discouraged if people aren't picking up on what you're trying to teach them. Everything will come back in spades. And that is exactly what's happened. The ripples have moved way out to the edge of the pond, and I am really happy about it. I've clung pretty closely to what I stated as my original goals and purposes. I've seen the fulfillment of things that I once thought impossible. It's a wonderful place for me to be now, having lived long enough to see so many huge positive shifts in the culture and in my own life.

*Constance-Marie Slater

Constance-Marie's lush annual Dressing for Pleasure Balls were the go-to event of the 1980s-1990s, drawing fetishists, cross-dressers, and sadomasochists the world over.

When I started out, I knew nothing. I had only discovered that kinkiness was inside me. As I stated in my book, *Kaleidoscope*, I was surprised when a male friend said, "You're such a bitch, you should be whipping ass." And I said, "I would never hurt anyone." And he said, "Hurting is not necessarily harming." So I went and I learned, and I discovered that I am a switch.

That's what was so wonderful with my husband, John: we were both switches for years, until he had his stroke and they put him on blood-thinners. After that, I couldn't cane him for fear of harming his skin, which had developed sores. So the playing stopped at that point in the marriage. The love was still there, as was the friendship and the business partnership.

After John died, my heart really went out of our fetish business. Too many people wanted me to listen to their problems and be their psychologist, and it was very wearying. My sister-in-law, Eileen, took over a lot of responsibilities after he died. So I said it was time. I was 67.

I'm in my 80s now and I am very happy. I live in Sullivan County in New York, in a lovely house on 60 acres of land, 40 of which are conserved forest. When I saw this home, I knew I wanted to live here until I die. Eileen now lives with me.

Presently, I don't consider myself an SMer because I haven't done anything in years. When I first moved up, I had someone who visited with me regularly. He loved to be caned. He was a golfer and said he played a better game after a caning. I hosted some lovely private parties for my old scene friends in the early years too, and their submissives came along, and we played on the deck, overlooking the woods. It was delightful. Still, I can't consider myself to be something if I'm not acting on it, and it's just not what I'm doing anymore. I would gladly still do SM because I really enjoyed playing, but it must be with the proper person and under the proper circumstances. I would love to find a man I could even go to dinner with. I haven't yet found anyone locally who is both single and intellectually suitable. I do miss the company of a man even though I'm very happy with my life choices.

When I closed on this house, there were a few lawyers who really irritated me. I told them that they really needed to be punished for the way they botched things. One of them said, "I do deserve to be punished, but not here." This intrigued me. But when I invited him to my house, he said, "Okay, but you won't tell anybody, right?" That was the end of that. I have no patience for duplicitous people.

But the lawyer who represented the seller is now my lawyer, and we've become socially friendly. He'll tease me when he sees me, saying, "Did you bring your whips and chains?" I know he spread word about me in our community. There is still so much shame about sex and prejudice against BDSM. I was afraid it would change perceptions of me but, apparently, it hasn't. I'm active in the Democratic Party, I'm active in local theatre, and I'm currently curating a show of my personal erotic art at a local non-profit community art gallery.

My involvement with the arts was a delightful twist for me. After I retired, one of the gentlemen who came to annual fetish events from Tennessee called and asked me to do a special, one-time auction event to raise money for their local theatre group. I suggested a professional auctioneer but he said it was too dull. They thought it would be a great idea to exhibit my personal collection of erotic art. So I took a bronze sculpture of Pan going down on a woman, which was valued at $6,000 and going up in value. I put my statue up and the opening bid was only $500. No one bid. As soon as we closed the auction, 3 different people came up to me and asked about it. They didn't want other people to know they might be interested in something sexy or erotic. I think it shows all the shame and fear that surrounds sex, especially unusual or kinky sex.

I don't know how many BDSMers keep playing into old age. I think that people change hormonally with age, and that it changes their sexual appetites, and that those changes can diminish their appetites for SM – unless they're masochistic or sadistic by nature. A sadist doesn't care what she does. I've seen sadists who are reckless and literally don't care if they cause harm. I steer people away from those types. A masochist just loves the pain and torture, and it has nothing to do with their sexuality in my opinion.

My best advice to people starting out is to know your Master or know your submissive. Have a conversation about limits, about what they want from the relationship. Some people really may not want more than a beating. Others may want the eroticism of a caring flogging. The submissive has to be satisfied: otherwise there is no game, no play. The submissive will not come back again, or feel engaged with the scene if they don't find pleasure with you.

*Morgan Lewis HMQ

Morgan is a beloved fixture of the NYC BDSM world, renowned for her career as a BDSM mentor and leadership role at Eulenspiegel.

BDSM has been the rounding out of my life. I didn't realize it was happening but I have become quite a mentor to people – they want to hear from me, they follow me on FetLife. Many, many men and women contact me for advice. I love it. BDSMers tend to be loving, kind people, who are incredibly intellectual. I'll tell you, I grew up in the church. I've spent my whole life around church people. But I discovered that whenever in my life I needed to rely on people, it was BDSM people who came to my rescue. It wasn't those Jesus people who did it.

I didn't learn to masturbate until I was 40! When I was working on my professional massage license, I got a temporary job at a massage parlor that turned out to be more like a whorehouse than a massage practice. I quickly figured out what was going on but I didn't care, I just did my thing and nobody made me do anything I didn't want to do. But I noticed one of the girls, every time she gave a guy a massage, she'd go take something out of a cabinet. I got curious so I asked what she was doing. She said, "Oh, I'm getting a vibrator so I can use it to masturbate to get turned on for sex with my client." I was so naïve, I was like, "WHAT?!!!" She laughed at me so hard, and told me, "You better go buy one for yourself." So I did, and I haven't been without one ever since! I have a Hitachi now, and if I wear it out, I just get a new one.

I never had problems about being into BDSM. I feel that our sexuality is ours to have: if it wasn't, we wouldn't have it. I always felt dominant, and I liked being a leader, so I was just myself when I got into the BDSM community. I ended up being the person answering the phone at TES when newbies called, and I was always the one at the door, welcoming newcomers, trying to put them at ease.

As a black woman, I don't know color. I grew up in a very integrated town in a very integrated neighborhood. We went to different churches but we were integrated at school. I didn't think about race much until I couldn't get working papers in my teen years, like all my white friends did. Then I learned. I really learned what it was to be black when I moved to New York.

I remember attending a panel in DC on Black people in the scene many years ago. At the time, Barry Douglas [*leather activist, former Chairman of the Gay Men's SM Alliance in NY*] said, "There's no reason to have a separate group for Black BDSMers. Don't be exclusive, be inclusive. SM is a small enough community, we don't need separatism." But other Black men on the panel pointed out that they couldn't necessarily afford the clothes, the events, the memberships that white BDSMers paid for. It was an economic reality and I understood the need. But I've never felt any racism within the scene. Never.

My life in the BDSM world gave me a chance to fully express myself and to put out what I feel about things. I've been teaching women to be dominant for the last 30 years. I know women have a hard time embracing a dominant role in this culture. So many of them are just playing at it. Worse, many are just not pushing back and will still accept abuse from men even when they are topping them in bed. I teach them to be dominant through and through, from the inside-out, not just how to satisfy men in the bedroom. I believe a dominant woman is a superior woman and I try to convey that to the women I educate.

I feel blessed to be recognized for my contributions. I was in New Mexico, visiting with Nancy Ava Miller, and there were lines of women who wanted to meet me and learn from me. That was amazing. I've made some incredible female friends over the years, especially on FetLife. I formed a women's group at my home about fifteen years. I started off with dominant women only, and called it The New York City Web. The members of the group started calling me Her Majesty the Queen to honor me, and suddenly I became known throughout the scene as HMQ. It's so funny because my sons tease me sometimes and call me that too. I feel so honored and so humbled. I feel so good that I've been a good girl, that people want to come to me and learn from me. What an amazing feeling that is!! It reinforces my belief that loving kindness brings everything.

My children have always known that my personal life is my business, and until they were of legal age, that their personal lives were mine. I told them my sex life is my business but it's not your business. I'm your mother, you're my child. My oldest son is a psychologist now and I told him I was going to an SM social. I invited him along, and he had a ball that night, talking to as many people as he could. He said, "Mom, that was one of the best parties I ever went to." He was just ordained as a minister, and he's in Uganda right now building schools and teaching people how to read and write.

A lot of people say that their hormones fade with age. I don't understand that. I'm not going to let my sexuality die. I was at the store the other day, and before you knew it, I was flirting with this young guy. It's not age: it depends on who you are, and how important sex is to you, and how much it is a part of you. Just because you get to be a certain age, your sex life doesn't have to die. I'm in my 80s, and I have a nurse's aide 7 days a week, but I am never going to stop having sex. You can't treat your sexuality like it's a separate part of you. It isn't.

I have new slaves all the time – they just want to be with me, some of them are just my slaves online. I have a new handsome man, he's a police officer with beautiful silver hair. He looks like a white statue. Just beautiful. And he loves taking off his clothes. So I said, "Take 'em off, baby, let's see." He loves having me just watch him.

Perhaps the most important thing I've learned about BDSM is to come to it with love in your heart. Never cram anything down anyone's throat that you don't believe yourself. If you come with love, it will all become beautiful. If you seek out your own sense of peace, you'll be surrounded by harmony. Self-love is the most cohesive and healing force in the world.

BDSMers 70+

*William Henkin

Psychologist, author, thinker and teacher, Dr. Henkin was a vital fixture in the San Francisco SM community. He gave us his interview a few short months before his death.

I came into the Community at a highly fortuitous time, in a highly fortunate place, San Francisco, and with a perfectly splendid partner, Sybil Holiday, who was herself a local luminary leatherwoman, and one of the hosts of the legendary Serpent Mountain mixed play parties. As a consequence I met and became friendly with some of the most remarkable, thoughtful, creative, and rigorous players in the scene within a few months. I went on to enjoy prolonged associations and friendships with several of them. There was also, at that time and in that place, a vibrant feeling of tribal family that thrilled me, and for which I am now deeply and gratefully nostalgic.

Communication – clean, clear, accurate, and timely – has been important to me for as long as I remember. One of my great delights when I entered the formal SM community in the 1980s lay in the disproportionately high number of people I met who shared this fetish. I was also quite familiar with concepts of personal responsibility and the like long before I came into the Community, but my participation wonderfully enhanced my understanding of consent in all matters, including the need for people to keep and honor our agreements, and not to change them unilaterally.

As a therapist serving the BDSM and other alternative communities for nearly 30 years I've seen a lot of people involved with different forms of erotic power play. For almost none has their participation in these activities been the presenting complaint or a significant contributor to the individual's pain and distress. When it has been, the person usually had not done sufficient homework and our initial work was devoted to education before anything else. I have seen BDSM difficulties in relationships, as with Dom/me-written slave contracts to which subs agreed but in which they never really participated enough to give informed consent. But, again, the issues have usually concerned unsatisfactory communication, thwarted expectations, and unfulfilled fantasies. When couples improve their communication skills, such problems dissipate.

If we take the concept of Top and bottom out of the equation – because in therapy there really is no Top or bottom, there are only two people matching needs, wants, and skill sets to attend to the concerns of one of them – then I can use a BDSM metaphor here even though it is only partly correct. Whether in SM or DS, it is important for the Top to maintain control so that the bottom can surrender or let go. Maintaining control does not mean the Top is not deeply engaged in a profoundly intimate process, it only means s/he is doing the necessary job so the scene can be fulfilling to both parties. Something related obtains in therapy, where the therapist must maintain control however deeply s/he is engaged, so that the client can delve deeply and process the material that comes up.

It's also true in BDSM, as I learned it, that a Top should never have the bottom do something the Top has not already tried out on her- or himself. Similarly in therapy I like to say that a therapist cannot go any deeper with a client than s/he has gone with her- or himself. I have always preferred to do long-term, deep, psychodynamic work, rather than short-term counseling or crisis interventions, though I've done my share of both. But my experience has shown me that it is the deep work that more often heals deep traumas, rather than fixing symptoms in bits and patches, partly because of the ways depth work relies on the client to engage with her or his own wounds in order for the healing to take place.

Though people often wish I could, in fact I cannot wave a magic wand and thereby repair damaged childhoods, disrupted relationships with people and things, or lost self-esteem, or make someone come to genuinely love his or her Self. As it happens, I do have a magic wand in my office, near my consultation chair, and it was my own 4½-year-old inner little boy, Master Billy Terror of the Universe, who taught me how to use it. He told me that if you really do the deep inner work that leads to encounters with all your Selves, including both those you think you like and those you think you don't like, and then wave the wand, you get that *ping!* of energy, and magic happens, healing happens, transformation happens. But if you wave a magic wand without doing the work, then you'll just be waving a stick around in the air.

I am aware of some of the more recent BDSM studies, particularly those that identify by research what players have known and talked about for decades. For example, one study recently documented ways in which some BDSM practices affect changes in blood flow to the brain that result in decreased stress and anxiety and greater calm and serenity. Sybil and I used to teach that the impact of a cane used by a skilled Top could focus both players' attentions exquisitely in the present. So the research data reflect exactly what players have long known to be a consequence of erotic energy exchange.

Another study found that some BDSM activities lead to states of consciousness similar to what some people achieve with meditation. This, too, is not news to experienced players. Indeed, as someone who has put in stints of meditation myself since the mid-1970s, I used to assert in many of the courses Sybil and I taught that, "I came for the sex and I stayed for the transcendence." Prolonged intense sensation, like prolonged attention to service, whether as a Top or as a bottom, opens the way to very deep states of being for those who want to follow such a path.

We did not do the research to give us statistically replicable results, but Sybil and I were far from alone in knowing these spiritually-oriented values of what we did. All that aside, however, I am a clinician, not a researcher, and while I'm pleased to know that the research community is finally learning what players have known since before my time, my concern is less with what the studies say and more with how the person in the room with me feels and thinks about what s/he is doing, and what the implications may be for her or his life, past, present, and future.

*Nancy Ava Miller

Pioneer and educator on professional female domination for almost 30 years, Nancy founded People Exchanging Power (PEP).

Before I discovered SM and particularly organizational SM, I felt that my entire life was a quest for more love, more sex, more attention, and more acceptability. After I got into SM it seemed like it was more of a spiritual experience. I melded with my partners in all new ways. The passion between us became so energetic and deep. That was new to me. BDSM really provided me with a sense of stability.

One big way it changed my relationships is that before getting involved in SM, I had tended to allow myself to not be taken seriously by men. I wouldn't say I let them abuse me, but I accepted a certain lack of respect for my needs and towards myself. After I got into SM, I started demanding more out of my relationships. I didn't become cruel or dictatorial but if I was going out on a date, there were new rules: he had to pick me up. If we were going out to dinner, he was going to pay. I gradually came to demand that men treat me the way I wanted to be treated. Not that more egalitarian relationships are wrong but they weren't right for me. I have had lovely relationships with guys who were broke, but I was done with deadbeats and takers. It wasn't just about money. I had a lovely slave in Washington who was a judge, and he used to sing me lullabies. He wasn't wealthy but he was doing well enough to fly me in. Another one didn't have any money but treated me so beautifully that I was content.

BDSM changed my view of sex. When I was young, blowjobs were coming into vogue and were considered really out there. I was married, and we had experimented with different positions. But I never realized there was a whole world out there of fetishes. It wasn't that I was closed minded, I just never really thought of anything beyond sexual intercourse. I wasn't even aware that I had already been privately engaged in SM because we didn't call it that. It was just something I joked about, like if I bumped into someone I might say, "Ooh, you really hurt me! You must be into SM." I had no idea you could actually live it. The biggest surprise for me was discovering that there was an entire counterculture out there that I wasn't even aware existed.

I've been exposed to so many unusual situations since my involvement in the scene. When I was growing up, any kind of varieties got criticized. Now that I am grown up, I've seen all kinds of happy unconventional people and witnessed all the incredible possibilities. Most people just see this stuff on television. So, for example, you may have heard about trans-sexed people but I was in a room full of naked trans-sexed people in various stages of transition and so what? They were just people. I've gotten to embrace all the realms of sexual possibilities in my own life. It has made me more accepting of life in general, and of other people's realities. I'm not more accepting of rape or murder, of course, but I welcome all the vibrant consensual possibilities. BDSM really provided me with a sense of stability.

Most of all, I'm not afraid to be myself anymore. If I'm waiting in line at the supermarket, and I get into chatting with someone, I'm not ashamed to tell them that I work in the sex industry if they ask what I do for a living. Especially now that I'm an older woman, people usually seem to be fascinated when I tell them my story, how I founded a group for perverts, and then founded a phone-domination service. If I sense they don't want to have a consensual conversation about it, though, I just say I'm a hypnotherapist or a writer. By the way, I really hate when prodoms say, "I'm not a whore!" What I hear is them trying to make pros (prostitutes) sound bad. The only difference between pros and prodoms is that prodoms may not have intercourse. Of course, some hookers may not have intercourse either. To me, it's all sex and we're all getting paid.

PEP (People Exchanging Power) was really born out of my own loneliness, desperation and horniness. I made trips to TES in New York, and learned everything I could about BDSM. When I started up the first group in Albuquerque, I modeled it on TES, using a support group modality as opposed to a sex club modality so people like me could feel comfortable. Once I had my own venue and group, I never felt lonely again! We would meet 3 times a week, so it felt like almost every night of my life was suddenly filled up – if it wasn't a meeting, it was talking to people and connecting with them. Founding PEP quenched my cravings for love and admiration. It really fed my ego to be so involved with others, serving a good cause. It also became easy to find sexual partners, which was a huge boon to my personal satisfaction.

I'm a child of the 1950s and 1960s, and I was a love-beads and flower-child person, very anti-money and anti-materialistic. Because I had a vision for an SM group, PEP suddenly turned me into a boss. So in addition to the emotional satisfaction, it led to me becoming fiscally responsible, and learning to pay attention to money and bookkeeping. That was amazing for me too.

When I married my slave, Barry, I thought it would be sex all the time and he would do everything I wanted. I guess I expected he would always be obedient, grateful and accommodating. He had a rebellious streak in him or reached a point where he was controlling and critical. That was a shock, that a submissive man would get so combative. Since then I've gained a lot of insight into human nature. When he got rude and manipulative, I learned to sway with it. I realized he wouldn't change and that I could endure it without turning into a bitch. I accept what it is and move on. He's flawed as we all are. I've accepted that he will never be my dream man because no one man ever could be.

If I want to stay married, I have to take the bad with the good, and keep my stride. I may be a dominant female, but I can't always get what I want. Or if I want it badly enough, there are better ways to get it than by nagging and yelling. There are kinder, more effective ways to work things out. I've had friends joke, "Oh if he's misbehaving, you should just spank him." But, honestly, I don't want to do BDSM when I'm pissed. I'd rather resolve the problem before I play.

I guess if I had one big message to convey, it isn't about BDSM really, but about loss. When I was younger, even small upsets overwhelmed me. Now, even at the worst of times, I can perceive some seed of potential goodness, some kernel of hope. Maybe it's a defense mechanism I developed after my grandson died. He had so many painful complications with his health that during the grieving process, the only thing that consoled me was knowing that had he lived, it would have been a terribly difficult life. So these days, when something bad or horrible happens, my mind automatically begins to seek out some tiny benefit that brings comfort. If I could go back in time, I would want to warn my younger self that loss is inevitable, so embrace and cherish the happy

moments that come your way. They are all precious.

*Gerrie Blum

Gerrie was involved in the formation of a range of metro NYC swing and BDSM groups, including one of the world's first online sex communities on the pre-Internet BBS system.

At the time of *Different Loving*, I was 54. I will be 78 in October 2015. I still live in the same apartment in Murray Hill and still work in Copiague on Long Island. I lost a year of my life to cancer in 2011 but have essentially recovered.

My partner Mitch Kessler and I have been together through it all since 1984. We made our first excursions into the "wonderful world of BDSM" together in 1986. The rest is history. I've "aged out" as a swinger but I am still a switch. I don't indulge in much activity outside my primary relationship with Mitch. My years among people in the Communities have led me to the conclusion that in most ways, we are pretty much just regular people, the same as everyone else. If there are any differences, it's that BDSMers try to deal openly with each other, even when there are power plays underlying our dynamics.

My best BDSM experience has been working in the business that Mitch Kessler and I founded over 25 years ago, Adam and Gillian's Sensual Whips and Toys. Our slogan is that we provide "implements of affection" to individuals worldwide. We make and sell what has grown to be the widest variety of paddles, floggers, straps, cats, canes and whips all made in one workshop. Over the years we have gained a reputation for quality and integrity, and we pride ourselves in making leather-ware of "heirloom quality." I still love going to work and talking to all the kinky people we deal with.

My other great experience was being included in the anthology, *Some Women* by Laura Antoniou. My contribution, "Somewhere to go, Someone to tell," described the kind of weekly meeting routine that we set up when I was an officer of the NYC Chapter of the National Leather Association. In short, every Monday night, if you arrived at a certain hamburger palace in midtown Manhattan, you could be sure of finding like-minded people in the downstairs dining room. It wasn't a "meat market" nor a meeting headed by a psychologist. You didn't have to explain yourself, or apologize for your thoughts and deeds. It was strictly a social gathering over coffee, or burgers, or sodas and the conversation was as likely to be about movies or sports or TV as it was about fetish clothing, or gear or clubs. The best part for me is that I've since seen the idea evolve into "the Munch" concept. Some people consider me to be "the mother of the munch" for my pioneering work in bringing kinky people together for low-key public gatherings.

My previous experience with organizational politics in conventional groups did not prepare me for the nature of the politics in the BDSM communities. (I always use that word in the plural ... we are not "one community" in many senses of the phrase.) Over time my circle became smaller and smaller, perhaps because I expected more of people than was realistic.

In general, I think I would advise my younger self to not take things so much to heart. One of the most powerful lessons I've learned from my life in kink is that no matter what your proclivities, there is always someone "kinkier than thou."

*Carter Stevens

Bon vivant and prolific porn producer, Carter is legendary for movies, magazines and parties catering to kinky tastes.

I was already pretty deep in the sex business when you interviewed me for *Different Loving*. It was through porn that I started to dabble in BDSM and discover I enjoyed the dom role. But your book was a nice prop to show a new sub. I could show her where I was quoted in a major work on the subject. It was a way to say, "See you can relax, now. I know what I'm doing." I know that's a cheap shot but I am a DOM (Dirty Old Man) and whatever gets me laid right?

My career in adult movies never disappointed me. I loved making films. I loved acting, producing, directing, writing, editing and any other job I could get involving motion picture production. My only surprise was coming to realize just how much I loved the fact that people were paying to watch ME do my thing on film. I discovered I was an exhibitionist!

My professional journey in BDSM was more rewarding than I could ever have dreamed it would be. The S&M NEWS took off from its very beginning and became the third largest BDSM paper in the country. As a result, my company grew and so did our publication list. We added fetish magazine after fetish magazine to our publications. *FOOTPRINTS* for foot fetishists, *SPANKS-A-LOT* for spankers, *COSMAPOLITAN DOMINA-TION* for Female Domination fans, plus a half a dozen other magazines including my favorites, which were two Male Dom mags titled *CHAINED* and *SLAVE*. They were my favorites because I shot 90% of all the photos in them during real (not simulated, pretend) bondage sessions.

By the time my heart blew up, my company was turning out two newspapers, two magazine issues, and several videos every month. But during the long recovery from my heart meltdown, the Internet came along. It killed my publishing empire as the BDSM community spread like wildfire across the Internet. You can't sell what everyone else is giving away for free. So I took the hint and retired.

The problem with being a rebel and an outlaw is that the pension plan SUCKS! If I had to do it all over, I'd say to myself SAVE YOUR MONEY. It won't last forever and we all get old. I'd also tell myself to slow down a little, go easy on the tequila, watch the cholesterol, but still never say no to a willing female.

*James

James was in a committed Mistress/slave relationship for over a decade and heavily involved in the BDSM world in the 1980-1990s.

When you first interviewed me, I thought I would be where I was forever. I was wrong. The change was both a surprise and a bitter disappointment, but the memory of where I was keeps me warm at night. Unhappily for both of us, my Mistress and I went separate ways. I met someone else and tried things out with her but it turned out not to be real enough, as I had come to understand this lifestyle. At present I am not active.

I could get sad about what happened but I prefer to remember a simply glorious period in which my psychic skin cracked open and I found and reveled in the life I had long dreamed about. I may not be there now, but I was there then and that is a life-long reward. Things happened.

As the song goes, I don't get around much anymore. I'm pretty reclusive. I am not active at present in the BDSM community and I have little interest in becoming active. I had everything I wanted and then I no longer had it. I tried to replicate something that could not be replicated and so I failed. I am not looking to do so again.

Looking back, if I was to give advice to the person I was 25 years ago, I'd say: Be honest with myself, be honest with others. Live in the present even if that means having memories and reminiscences of the past while in the present. Be kind to others whenever possible. Don't assume people are being mean when they're only being ignorant. As Bob Dylan wrote, "Don't go mistaking Paradise for that home across the road."

BDSMers 60+

*Mitch Kessler

Founder of SM groups, former publisher and editor of SM magazines, and activist, Mitch now devotes his energy to running his BDSM toy company.

When "Youth does at last decay," things do change. I'm 67 years old now. In 1991, based on my sexual behavior, I was bisexual. Certainly my political sympathy was entirely with what today we call the LGBT community. But with the passage of time, the whitening of the beard, and the spreading of the paunch... Well, to be a "Bear" is one thing, but "Santa" is not who the men I found attractive found attractive in return. And who can blame them? So, over time, the "bisexual" became more theoretical, and, with one thing and another I found myself investing more time and energy in my dyadic relationship... leaving less time for either casual encounters or public play.

"Polyfidelity" is a whole other topic. Suffice to say, it was a decidedly minority opinion for most kinksters during the 20th century. Poly was not condemned per se, but not often practiced successfully, over any long period of time. The strong dominant identity is maybe a little more interesting. THAT was always more legend than fact. In "the Scene" (before we called it The Community) fat girls got respect, bisexuals were tolerated as "exotics" (and with more goodwill than in some parts of the Gay and Lesbian Community), but male submissives were regarded in much the same light as squeegee men and busboys.

At the time, I was trying to organize a Pansexual alternative organization to TES. I believed that my credibility as an organizer/Community Leader depended on my "He Who Tops Tops" reputation. And while I might occasionally bottom in public clubs, it was NEVER with a glossy-flossy Dominatrix-Ma'am – it was ALWAYS with a deferential entourage in attendance.

My BDSM business, ASWGT [ed-Adam's Sensual Whips and Gillian's Toys], is still doing quite well. We're not one of the major players in the BDSM Gear trade but we have a loyal following who appreciate our craftsmanship and design, and they seem to keep recommending us to others.

For me, the biggest surprise AND disappointment was the banality and cronyism of the organizational politics in The Scene. Is it different from insider cliques at a Country Club or any House of Worship? No. But from that realization sprang both the surprise and the disappointment. If there is a piece of advice my 'now self' would give to my 'then self' it would be, "Where Community Affairs are concerned... go along to get along."

I suppose the public collaring of my boi and then her private release, were the high points of my journey. In retrospect, I was enacting Shakespeare's Tempest with myself as Prospero. For a while I ruled benevolently over my little island kingdom (the NYC Chapter of the National Leather Association) and enjoyed the pomp and deference due an exiled Duke of Milan... and then came the time at which the circle had to close so I drowned my Book, broke my Staff, and freed my Ariel. Since much of my involvement with The Scene had been fueled by a desire for authenticity or to achieve some higher ground, this grand renunciation was real, it was important – and it did set me free. But it was also the beginning for me of true exile.

In general: people, myself included, are people, and their sexual signatures reflect who they are – but only approximately. I found the distinction between BDSM and real life wasn't nearly as significant or interesting as I might wish for. For me, the idea that personal relationships involved power exchanges came as no surprise. That some of us would dramatize that fact with play was just a wonderful icing on the cake. My mentor in The Scene, Brenda Howard [*noted bisexual advocate and activist*] once said, "BDSM makes sex so complicated... and that's why we like it." Which, so far as it goes, turned out to be quite true.

I think that powerful lessons come in life when you're ready to learn them. In the end, as long as "Kinky" is even remotely Safe Sane and/or Consensual, it is not so very different than any other philosophy, affiliation or pastime.

*Alexis deVille

Trans woman, professional dominatrix and fetish aficionado, Alexis has over four decades of experience in the BDSM world.

I'm bisexual and transgendered, living as a female 90% of time. I am an IT & Robotics Consultant. Nearly all of my clients know me now as a woman, but some of the old guard clients still only know me as a male. It's not easy to maintain that male identity anymore.

I am in the same open relationship with my long-time partner and female lover as when I was interviewed for the first book. I'm 67 and we've been together for 45 years. We really care for each other. We still enjoy a good sex life. I've always been very oral. She used to visit a lot of clubs with me in the past, all the alternate clubs. I'd dress club style and she dressed more conservatively. Eventually, she didn't want to come along, while I was going more and more. She's perfectly okay with me going out on my own. We're together for life.

I was attending a study meeting once, as a volunteer for research on transsexualism. The doctor there came up to me afterwards and said that I was the most well-adjusted, well-balanced transsexual she had ever met. That was funny but sweet. I now have natural boobs, size 36 C. No implants, just hormones. I got some injectables in Mexico, and have used other hormones, and now they look like absolutely natural breasts. Oddly, taking estrogen has made me more horny.

These days, I am mostly into very generous submissive men and the odd straight guy not into kinky. I meet them when I'm traveling, or sometimes through work. They hit on me, LOL! It's great how much action I still get. I still do some pro Dominatrix work because that helps to keep me in heels and fetish wear! I only have sex with very select partners – either because we've formed special relationships or they are former clients who I became attached to. I've ordered some to remain in chastity while they are away from me. If their chastity is broken when I see them, then sex is off the table. But I do enjoy feeling someone I care about coming inside me.

I've been going to fetish events most of my adult life. I only had one scary experience in all these years. I was dominating someone in a fantasy scenario when he suddenly turned the tables on me. He was bigger than me, so it was intimidating. But I know my way around men. It wasn't hard to convince him that I wanted to be submissive to him, and wanted to caress his balls. It was easy for me to regain control once his balls were in my hand! I gave them a rough twist and then I was right back in control. That was my first and only experience with someone who tried to turn the tables. It was a little frightening, I must say.

Everyone's a little sadistic in the role of dominant but I would say stay away from pathological sadists. I've seen dominatrices beat their submissives until they could barely walk. People who are submissive should stay away from true sadists who want to break their limits. I watched a professional dominatrix at Pandora's Box go beyond a limit and ignore safe words. That's not acceptable. I always play safely and abide by safe words.

What I've really learned from my life in BDSM is that some of the nicest and smartest folks are like ME and into Kinky! Really some of the nicest people I've ever met, extremely intelligent people, whether or not they had great professions. I'm very happy with my choices. My sex life is a blast!

*Sybil Holiday

Popular BDSM teacher, lecturer and former professional dominatrix, Sybil had to step back from her career because of a disability.

When I was first interviewed in 1991 I was 42 years old, considered myself a leatherwoman, and was very involved in the leather community in San Francisco. That initial interview was also conducted under my prodomme name, M. Cybelle, and today this one is under my private name, Sybil Holiday. Now, at age 66, I wouldn't call myself socially a leatherwoman as my relationship to the current leather community is very different than the one I had with the group of folks I encountered in 1980.

But I have always had an alpha personality; it was simply brought to the surface, and then honed in that world. I should also point out that I don't use the term BDSM. For me, my sexual and social nature is still described by the terms that existed when I started out in 1980; SM, leather sex, and Top and bottom. In 1984 the term D/s (dominance/submission) were created, and I found they were applicable to my way of being in charge as it isn't really a role for me, it is an authentic way of being.

BDSM is a huge, overlapping term that holds no real meaning for me, and I'm also unhappy that the D/s in the middle of those overlapping initials gets lost *a lot*. I haven't played either privately or professionally since 2005, but if I did privately today it still would be D/s, energy-based SM, and teaching service from a spiritual perspective.

I miss the structure that I encountered in the gay leather scene. Through those experiences with leathermen and leatherwomen I learned to process pain, get high on endorphins from a decent cathartic flogging, I learned about erotic energy and how to exchange it, and I learned to actually surrender control and authority. I believe these personal experiences, and the knowledge gained, of both mind and body, is what made me such an in-tune whip-mistress and Domina.

My life in this world has taught me some important lessons. Before I found leather and topping, I had been covert about my sexual needs. I didn't realize it at the time but I never directly asked for what I wanted sexually. I couldn't verbalize my desires, I would just let a partner know if I liked something by sound and movement, and I'd go completely still and quiet if I didn't. But I never spoke directly about it, I couldn't say, "A little more to the left, and slower." With SM and being a Top it was a given that I was supposed to give direction and even to require that my sexual needs get cared for first. I'd never done that before, even as an outrageous stripper and hippie who was into equality. It was incredibly empowering.

I also learned how a fetish can be extraordinarily specific. I have average feet with a nice high arch BUT my toenails are a little odd, some curve straight upward. In the beginning I encountered a few foot fetishists who told me my feet weren't pretty enough for them to worship. I knew my feet weren't perfect, but I didn't realize how specific a fetish could be until clients rejected my feet! So after that I never offered foot worship. The closest I could do was shoe and boot worship. Professionally, I owned over 300 pairs of shoes and boots whose soles never touched pavement.

In the spring of 1988 I met the love of my life. Our foundational meeting was as Mistress and submissive, and a year and a day later we got hand-fasted, with a ritual where I declared him my slave, and he got a ritual piercing. We had 18 months of bliss and then in 1989 I developed such significant and severe back pain issues that my whole life changed, and has never been the same. Unfortunately I was misdiagnosed for ten months. I finally got a correct diagnosis and treatment in 1990, but my sex drive didn't return. By 1991 we were no longer really participating as Mistress and slave. My sex drive didn't return until winter 1994. That was the last time we tried to play. By then he couldn't bottom to me. We never did D/s or SM again after that. In 1995 we performed a formal ritual together: we buried a box containing the collars he'd worn for me, and some special items, under a Redwood tree in northern California. We left a note with it asking that if someone found it to not open or disturb the contents as there was nothing of intrinsic value in the box, only grief.

For the next three years the relationship continued as people who deeply love each other but aren't being sexual. For a while I thought, it will be okay, I have other slaves for my SM jollies. We even tried vanilla sex, but that didn't work as neither one of us are vanilla. However he couldn't get what he *needed* and that was emotionally devastating for us both. We both grieved the passing of that part of our relationship though our love for each other was as powerful as ever. As I love with an open hand, we agreed he could meet and bottom to other dominant women as long as I felt okay about them.

In the spring of 1997 a dominant woman who had been seeing him for some time wanted to own him. As we were engaged I told him if he needed that, okay, but I could not be engaged to a man who was owned by another woman. We did another ritual ending our engagement, and I asked that we not talk for a month. During that time I did some serious inner work of disconnecting and letting go of our relationship completely, and making myself fall out of love.

After we separated, we both moved on in separate ways. We stopped communicating regularly because it was too painful for us both. I kept busy and life was okay. Not amazingly wonderful but certainly not awful. I formed a long-term relationship with my leathergirl. Around 2007 his relationship with his new Mistress changed, and he felt he wasn't getting the support he needed at a time of personal crisis. As he came to new awakenings about that relationship and himself, he reached out to me again, and we started talking every day. After that, we stayed best friends. We were talking in a different way from our old D/s interaction but felt as close as ever. I was his Spiritual advisor. In a sense, we fell back in love. It wasn't sexual but the love and deep friendship survived 26 years, until his death last year.

I kept teaching and playing until 2005, when the progressive degenerative disk and bone disorder that dramatically changed my life in 1989 flared up again, only much, much worse this time. I was doing a class one weekend when the physical agony was so great that I could not stay focused. That was the moment I decided to end my BDSM teaching career and stop seeing all clients. In 2010 I got a more effective medicine. Still, it took four years to recover from pain exhaustion. I use a wheelchair now since it is a progressive disorder. I also had a few bad experiences that made me wish to distance myself from the leather part of the kink community here in San Francisco, and from 2010 until 2014 I didn't even wear leather clothing; all were folded and put away in a bottom drawer.

The most powerful life lesson I've learned throughout it all is that nothing is guaranteed. Even if someone promises to be your slave for life, it's still not guaranteed. I would've thought nothing could separate my partner and me. I've learned that everything can change, and come and go and return and go again; people, situations, health, things, beliefs, one's sexuality, and so much more. And so I've learned that the only thing that is guaranteed is my essence; not my body, not my mind, but my heart. AND that I will survive and triumph through adversity. Because really, what other choice is there?

Chrissy B.

Chrissy is a transwoman in transition, though she has been aware of her true gender identity since early youth.

I wouldn't say BDSM has shaped either my life or my view of relationships. It's the opposite. Throughout my life BDSM has been the lens through which I see the world and the framework in which I've lived.

The biggest disappointment without question has been the transitory nature of some individuals' interest and acceptance. While they seemed to enjoy the power exchange dynamic, it turned out to be a passing fantasy, while the reality of a negotiated, full time relationship was more than they could handle. The biggest positive, on the other hand, has been making dynamic, vital connections with people who are actually in touch with their core spirituality and are committed to living their truths.

My public and family life until recently has always been quite vanilla. What has changed in the past year is that I've come out as trans, and in the process have finally cultivated a circle of friends who accept me fully in both my authentic gender and kink identity. In doing so they have reinforced my confidence about transitioning. I'm truly comfortable around them and see them as people who are in touch with their own desires, their gender identities and their personalities, and as friends who are able to clearly define themselves as being somewhere on the gender and/or D/S spectra. Whether they're overtly expressing their D/S persona at any particular time is a different issue.

Some of my most intense experiences actually came early in my exploration, somewhere in the early 1970s. Her scene name was Mademoiselle DuPont, and I've always wondered what became of her – after our third or fourth meeting she simply disappeared. She was the first woman who (with the help of her slave girl) stripped me of every hair below my eyebrows and showed me that I would and should become a pleasing and submissive girl.

Another highlight for me was attending the early Eulenspiegel Society parties in New York. There was a kinky couple who I met at one of the parties and who brought me to later events, and then used me as a party favor for their guests and friends. What made those experiences great was the freedom from making decisions. Once I consented to the role, I surrendered to it and allowed myself to be used as an object of pleasure and lust by others. That sense of surrender fulfilled some deep and delicious craving inside me... it's a sensation I seek out and relish to this day.

My BDSM journey itself has been unpredictable, which is precisely what I should have expected, even if I didn't at the beginning. I think I first realized that I was more a girl than a boy when I was 8, though I couldn't have articulated it clearly back then. It took a few more years for me to identify as a submissive. And this year, at the age of 65, for the first time I marched as a very proud woman in the New York City Pride Parade. I couldn't believe how emotional and thrilling that experience was.

The most powerful lesson I've learned from life as a kinky, transgendered person is that we're all different but we're all the same. Our kinks vary by person, and few are truly identical. But at our core we're all seeking fulfillment on a very deep level. Some of us are simply more honest about it than others.

*Cléo Dubois

Legendary professional sadist, spiritual voyageur and inspirational educator, Cleo is devoted to helping new generations of sexual adventurers find their own paths.

Carrying the torch of consensual sadomasochism is my life's work and pleasure. With maturity comes a deeper understanding of what really matters: self-acceptance, healing, satisfying erotic exchanges, the value of human connection and community.

Over the years, I have become a skilled BDSM educator, a caring sadist, versatile player and shamanic ritualist. I first met Fakir in 1983 at a Janus [*ed. - Society of Janus in San Francisco*] meeting. Intrigued, I attended his esoteric programs. Body rites and spirit were obviously his path. In 1987, I asked him to pierce me and stitch balls and bells on my upper back and chest like he had done. I needed to shake my grief in a ceremony of my own. It was my first "Ball Dance," embracing the sensations the pierced weights added to my dancing, crying, screaming for my beloved dead. That day I saw Fakir's gentle side. I was charmed. In 1988, I asked him for a date. Two years later, we tied the BIG knot! In a magnificent redwood grove in Northern California. A large circle of kinksters, Shamans and Leather Faeries blessed our union. Missing was Cynthia Slater, the founder of Janus. AIDS took her the previous fall.

To this day, Fakir and I work as a team offering hook pulls and suspension rituals. So I'd call BDSM/Fetish "total impact," a real life changer for me. We are life partners, still living together and loving each other. Of course, we continue working on our relationship. As we age, we grow closer and more tender, more accepting of our differences. In the past 10 years we have formed a leather family with another kinky couple and a bi-male lover. Queer in spirit, we belong to a tribe of folks of mixed sexual orientations and gender with whom we continue to share our ritual energies.

Shortly after *Different Loving* was published, Fakir and I traveled to Malaysia where I was taken (psychically connected) by Kali, the fiery spirit Mother archetype I serve. Namaste. Working with archetypes in BDSM, rather than just roles, has deepened my experiences and enriched my ability to lead others on their kinky path. By 2000, I had become a sought-after Leather presenter. To reach out further, I made my first docu-film, "The Pain Game," about connected BDSM play. Recognized for its authenticity by the SSSS [*Society for the Scientific Study of Sex*], it continues to inform folks in the US and Europe and be part of sex-ed classes. My bondage docu-film, "Tie Me Up," followed in 2002, combining rope tips with play dynamics. While I also offer video instruction online at Kink Academy and a bit at Kink.com, nothing surpasses the value of mentoring, in person, in real time. My professional practice today is focused on coaching Dominants and their partners who seek to illuminate their dark desires with mutually satisfying BDSM play.

My journey has never been about expectations, it's about discoveries! When I think back, I am amazed at how much I learned about humanity and sexuality from my twenty years in professional dominance and being in community. I am delighted that I am invited to visit many places as a BDSM educator and ritualist. Not only in the US, but also Paris, Tokyo, Osaka, Lisbon, London, Copenhagen, Penang, and Mexico City. That is, of course, one of the plusses of also being Fakir's wife!

Recently I have presented to groups I did not think were open to kink! While I sometimes consider it "kink lite," I nonetheless do my very best to honor the pioneers, Leathermen and Leatherwomen I had the privilege to learn from and play with. I still believe in the magic of SM! It is all about deeply connecting, building energy and the strong bonds we form in the process. I love to guide couples in the privacy of my dungeon and to witness their *aha* moments. The trust they put in me is a gift I cherish and honor. Along with my friend Eve Minax [*respected BDSM educator and activist*], my Academy of SM Arts offers weekend

Intensives for players of all genders as well as ethical training for Professional Dominas.

The mainstream's new-found tolerance of the alternative lifestyles of the radically sexual (us) is a somewhat mixed blessing. Tolerance is not acceptance. I wrote articles, I participated in many psychological surveys assessing our sanity, always advocating acceptance. So, the shameless joy of kink these newbies embody surprises me! We, as a Judeo-Christian society, seem to have finally turned a page. And I am learning to enjoy the fruits that grew from our persistent labor as elders in the leather/kink community.

As a Domina I learned that everyone needs to belong, to be accepted, to have their fetish respected. Shame and isolation does not work for anyone. Embodying my own erotic archetypes, expressing my caring sadism as well as experiencing safe surrender in my bottom masochistic headspace has allowed me to reclaim my sexuality. In fact, it has also given me a new appreciation of vanilla lovemaking.

I am very grateful to have been interviewed for *Different Loving*. It is the True "Fifty Shades of Kink," a ground-breaking book that stands the test of time. A woman who could be my adult daughter thanked me recently, adding that my interview in *Different Loving* changed her life. It also brought many clients to my little dungeon. Merci beaucoup! On Dec. 1st, 2012, I started blogging, an inspiring challenge since English is my second language. I enjoy sharing my true stories and now I am seriously considering writing my autobiography.

When I came out I was fearless, passionate and quite a bit too fiery! I lived on the edge. I needed to learn to respect boundaries and set my own. I know I scared more than a few! From my mistakes I have learned to be sensitive to limits and aware of the surprise landmines some kinky explorations can trigger. My compassion has grown. Like a good French wine I have mellowed.

As Ram Dass says, "there are many paths to the top of the mountain but from the top the view is the same." The path of BDSM is really about connection, sexual energy and compassion. Many trusted me with their dark erotic secrets and gave me permission – or begged me – to play with them. My advice to those just discovering their sadistic turn-ons is that toys are great, but energy is more important. Take a breath. Take another. Now, slow down, connect and go for the energy! It's a loop; you send it out and your bottom sends it back to you. Stay connected!

*Dian Hanson

Dian Hanson has been creating high-quality vehicles for fetish art and eroticism for over 30 years, from books and magazines to curated art shows.

Wow, 1991 was a lifetime ago. *Leg Show* magazine was in its ascendance at that time. It continued to grow and evolve until 1997, reaching a peak readership of 200,000 a month, with three foreign editions (German, French and Spanish). After '97 sales inched downwards as the Internet took over. In 2000 my beloved publisher, George Mavety, who made my career by giving me complete editorial freedom, died suddenly. The company struggled on for a year, with horrible mismanagement and then a very disreputable coalition took control. I hated to leave my loyal fans, but knew I had to get out.

I left the first week of September 2001, thereby missing the World Trade Center destruction a mile south of our offices. Fortunately, my most loyal fan was Benedikt Taschen, whose publishing company was steadily growing as magazine publishing was declining. He'd wanted me to head his Sexy Book division for several years, and I called him up and said, "OK, I'm ready." I became TASCHEN's Sexy Book editor in November 2001, still the best job title ever.

In the years since I've written and edited over 60 books, including the six volume *History of Men's Magazines*, five volume "body parts" series, starting with *The Big Book of Breasts*, then *The Big Penis Book*, *The Big Book of Legs*, *The Big Butt Book* and finally *The Big Book of Pussy*, *Vanessa del Rio: Fifty Years of Slightly Slutty Behavior*, *Tom of Finland*

XXL, *Terryworld*, *Psychedelic Sex*, and out soon, *Lesbians for Men*, an historical overview of men's fascination with lesbian sex acts.

Working with these men, and for these men – since all my books and magazines have been in the service of sexual satisfaction – has broadened my base of knowledge about all forms of sexuality, increased my well of empathy, and made my diverse knowledge a big hit at dinner parties. It has not altered my basic sexuality, which is uninhibited, but not particularly unusual.

I'm now 64 years old, and I'll be celebrating 19 years with my husband, author Geoffrey Nicholson, in November 2015. He's not the one I was with in 1991, but you can see I'm still a fan of long-term relationships.

I'm a high school dropout, so most of my education came from what I saw, read, and heard while first making my magazines, and now making my books. I research every topic extensively, so each new title offers the opportunity to pick up new information that impacts my life view – as does the knowledge I gain. For example, I learned daily from readers' letters when I was making magazines. The first lasting lesson was that men are just as romantically inclined as women. I expected letters to a sex magazine to be about sex, but fantasies of love and yearnings for relationships with the women in the magazines were just as common. So many men also wrote about their wives with obvious pride and affection.

I heard from men whose fetishes I knew would prevent them from forming satisfying relationships, like the guy who was only aroused by seeing women step on a wax effigy of himself, or the man who felt compelled to collect and drink women's sputum while they watched in disgust. I couldn't help them find love, but I could hear their confessions without freaking out, and offer kind words. To me, they were just humans seeking love like any other.

I also heard from men who gained the courage to open up to their partners by sharing *Leg Show* with them and then found acceptance. The most gratifying of these was a man who called me the morning of his wedding to tell me that my advice had given him the courage to tell his girlfriend he was a foot fetishist. He had never expressed his fetish in any way but masturbatory fantasy. She asked him to show her what he found pleasurable, and the sharing deepened their bond and led to marriage, so he had to call and tell me. We were both in tears.

After all these years so many men are still in the closet, either not out to their wives, or their wives have rejected that part of their sexuality and they've diverted it to professionals. It's sad but predictable that male fetishists – and fetishists are still mostly male – 20 years on still haven't found the holy grail of females with corresponding tastes, since there simply aren't, say, a pool of women fantasizing about men sniffing their feet. There are much greater commercial opportunities for satisfaction, though, thanks to the Internet. Steve Savage puts on regular FootNight parties in Los Angeles, San Diego, Toronto, Las Vegas, and Detroit, where men pay a $65 entrance fee for the opportunity to engage the feet of attractive women, many of them porn performers. The girls negotiate fees for various acts of foot worship with each man, in public or private, but for nothing beyond that. It's not always reciprocal lust, but some women really enjoy the worship, and in general they have a good time and treat the men well, and many have built strong followings. Perhaps as important as the sexual outlet, it gives the guys a chance to meet other fetishists in a bonding, shame-free atmosphere. A recent party in Los Angeles featured 54 young women with a variety of foot sizes and shapes.

I was saying to a friend recently that the fetish liberation movement is a long way off. Today, as I write this, all laws against same-sex marriage were declared unconstitutional, with President Obama declaring, "Love is love." The current transgender rights movement is also receiving strong support in the media and the academic world, but it's hard to imagine these same groups getting behind a sexual minority made up almost exclusively of men united by interests most often expressed through solitary masturbation. True fetish and partialism – the substitution of non-sexual body parts for the genitals – has always been romantically alienating. People feel unloved when their partners prefer their panties, socks or feet to their vaginas or penises, and fetishists most suffer this stigma. Right or wrong, we judge by lovability. The gay marriage struggle succeeded through its connection to love. But who stands beside the foot or panty fetishist? Fetish seems comical, at best, and threatening at its most misunderstood. Most wives and girlfriends would still just rather the guy keep it in the closet.

When I began doing *Leg Show* I saw the loneliness and pain suffered by men who believed their sexuality was abnormal. No one wanted to be a pervert. Many had spent years on the couch trying to rid themselves of perversion, yet I never received a single letter saying therapy cured them. Some had even resorted to hormonal suppression of their sex drives, which blunted, but did not change, their tastes. I developed a deep sympathy for these stricken souls and used *Leg Show* as a platform for understanding and education, not to eliminate their imbedded orientation, but to accept and enjoy it, since there really is no escape from who you are.

My best advice to newcomers is to explore it through fantasy first, to discover the full scope of your particular sexuality. Approach the Internet with caution. Don't reveal yourself to casual sex partners, but don't wait so long to divulge what you need in an established relationship either. It's tempting to wait until you've made the person love you to tell them your secret, but they'll then feel tricked and manipulated. Either that, or your fear of rejection will lock you in the closet forever. Bring it up casually, as if it's no big deal, when you both realize you like each other, but long before you're planning the wedding.

Patrick Mulcahey

Sought-after speaker and popular BDSM writer, Patrick is one of the BDSM's world's most recognized and esteemed leaders and thinkers.

The "organized scene" is hard to find if, A) you don't know what it looks like, and B) you don't know what it's for. I went to leather bars and small play gatherings (not much resembling what we call "parties" now) way back in the 1970s. I'm not antisocial, but I might be a little mulish. Organized activities, teams, outings, being given duties and told what to do – I just was never that kind of joiner. I'm fully aware my contrarian ways border on the absurd. I remember going to smoking cessation programs where I'd listen to the speakers and think, "Fuck you! I'll smoke if I want to!"

The 1980s for me were a detour into AIDS activism and watching my friends die. I found IML [*International Mr. Leather Contest*] in the early 1990s, but only the hot sex phenomenon; I didn't attend any part of the contest for another ten or twelve years. It was all about the action then, for me, and the action was not to be found in theaters, auditoriums, or meeting rooms.

I didn't show up on a regular basis for any group or event until I figured out it was easier to find play partners through the 15 Association [*SM/BD gay leather group in San Francisco*] than on my own. That would've been 2003 or 2004. I have uncertain recollections of being at a handful of their parties in the 1990s as a guest, maybe at their big Dore Alley or Folsom parties, but back then I really had no sense of the club or of its identity. My play otherwise was entirely private, always an adventure, never lasting very long with any one partner. There was a lot I wasn't bringing to the table, I realize now.

I had a vanilla partner at home and thought of my draw to leather as only an itch to scratch. When I first broke out the cuffs with my ex back in 1985, he piped right up: "Oh, no. If you want *that*, you'll have to find it somewhere else." It was the 80s, it was the end of the world, we all thought we were dying, and here was a man who loved me, just not my rope and restraints. So I said okay. I didn't know myself very well and ended up breaking his heart because of it.

That BDSM was just an occasional fancy was a lie I was telling myself, and that was what had to change before I could start showing up in public and semi-public group settings with guys who accepted me and knew me by name, to whom consequently I had a kind of commitment to be the same person one month to the next. I started building social capital where I hadn't understood there was anything but the sexual to pursue. The idea that friends, strangers, clubs, contest organizers, bar owners worked together to create these intensely hot sexual environments I was seeking out had somehow not occurred to me until then.

I'm not big on "identifying." Now, I am not one of those "labels are meaningless" people either. They are meaningful when employed with care and precision; demographic study, which can be meaningful too, relies on such social and sexual categories. Since age nineteen, I have been checking the "male" and "gay" boxes on surveys, and by the time it dawned on me that it might be helpful to have a kink identity, I decided on "bondage Top." Nowadays, though, hokey as it sounds, I identify by my name. I wonder if what you have called the organized scene is transitional for most of us. It was invaluable to me when I found it, but I don't know how long I'll stay connected to it.

"Identifying" is about explaining yourself to other people: my project is about explaining me to me. People trying to figure me out from what they can see of my relationship will peg me as "Dominant" and, what tends to surprise them, as "monogamous." It surprised me too. I have very few friends in sexually exclusive relationships, as far as I know, and I never made any big decision to be monogamous myself. It turns out to be a little decision you make every day: should I pursue this new possibility, or just go home? I keep going home. But I don't consider being monogamous an "identity." It's just the form this specific relationship assumed.

Occasionally people try to hang the "Master" tag on me and I have to object. I don't know what anyone but my husband/slave could mean by calling me Master. I joke that people can call me Master Patrick the day Race Bannon lets people call him Master Race. I will also say that inwardly I am faithful to the designation "leather." To be honest, I don't think it means much anymore, but that's what it was called when I found it.

For me, the journey's been all about self-knowledge. Even after coming out as gay (and my coming out story is of the traumatic variety), I was still leading my life for the benefit of other people, not me. Leather began to show me how to remedy that.

What we call normality is a feeling you're in a movie everyone is watching, so you goddamn better get it right. Once you stop believing (or caring) that you're being watched and start looking inside, you can get on to more serious things. There's a quality of attention you have to pay to yourself and to your partner in BDSM that's rare, and revelatory. I kept wanting more of it. I don't mean more of the sensations. If sex is mostly about what's happening in your head, BDSM is about making what's happening in your head happen before your eyes. Carefully, so you don't get lost, or if you do, so you can find your way back.

And even once we begin, it takes years to get to what is ground-floor real in us. We adopt cartoon roles and costumes to suit them: we're *dark*, we're *bad*, we're *nasty*, we're *insatiable*, we're *rebels*. But being badder, darker, more insatiable, more rebellious is still to define yourself by comparison to some conventional standard. With a little luck, though, one of those poses will jolt you out of it. That's what happened to me. I was in the middle of an elaborate, days-long roleplay scene, and it hit me like a bolt of lightning: the man I thought I was playing was real, was me. It was everything else in my life that was fake.

So one of my surprises was how inauthentic people can be when they're determined to be "authentic." And I don't exempt myself from the charge. The off-the-rack roles we absorb from the kinkosphere or pornosphere and impose on each other are obstacles to solid relationships. The strain of taking on those poses (the groveling slave, the imperious Dom, etc.) can mask, even doom, whatever might be the real possibilities between us. We play: "I'm a lock, you're a key – we must be a fit." Yet how else can we start, lacking in experience as we are? We don't learn about kink dating or leather relationships in adolescence. The dearth of role models doesn't help. There may be more of us "out" in leather and kink these days, but how many kink relationships can you observe close-up? Mostly they hum along under the radar.

It also surprised me when I detected my desires were changing. I imagine it happens to everyone, but I wasn't prepared for the slow realization that what I desired was *leading* me to something else, something I wanted even more but didn't know how to name. I don't actually feel "kinky" anymore. Does that qualify as a surprise? I don't mean that what turns me on has changed (though it has, some). I mean the way I think and feel about it.

My husband Patrick and I met in March of 2007 on Recon, an online site for kinky gay men, leather-oriented originally, then blossoming into other flavors. Neither of us was using it as a hookup site at the time. I liked it for chatting with leather friends across the country and internationally. We spent a month negotiating a first meeting. We were both pretty savvy. I liked how insistent he was on both his submissive nature and on being treated with respect. This was not some guy spinning a fantasy who would beat off and disconnect. We discovered we knew all the same people, had been in the same places at the same time, but had just never met.

He was different from anyone ever. That's when I understood my desire was leading me to something new. It led me to him. And he keeps leading me to me. It took us almost a year to figure out that the Master-and-slave archetype suited us well. Which, as I say, doesn't feel "kinky" to me. That same archetype was the design of all marriages for centuries. And now somehow it's weird?

The last thing I thought I would ever want was to be married. Our dynamic means that he lives in a state of extreme dependency on me, so I wanted all possible legal protections for him, should anything happen to me. But after spending a few thousand dollars on attorneys and trusts and wills and other documents, I had to accept that the most complete protection was marriage. I didn't think about the emotional and psychological aspects of being married until after it happened.

One consequence of our being married that tends to make people gasp or laugh: when I decided we'd have a wedding after all, Patrick asked if he could take my last name. Which sounded crazy to me, for about twenty seconds. So now we are both me: Patrick Mulcahey.

He and I have been through the fire together. The details are private and would anyway fail to convey the highest highs and lowest lows of both our lives. I'm as much at ease with him now as when I'm alone. Being with him *feels* like being alone, in the sense of being with myself. Guy Baldwin [*SM author and activist, inductee in the Leather Hall of Fame*] married us! And has made it very clear, vocally, in that Guy Baldwin voice, that any bond so forged by him is to be considered indissoluble.

Race Bannon

A proud public face of BDSM and LGBT activism since the 1980s, Race is an indefatigable innovator, creator, author, and leader in the leather/BDSM communities.

In 1973, I was 18, living in Chicago and going to gay men's leather bars (underage at the time per their local liquor laws). I worked in one of the kinkier bars as a bartender too. So I was knee deep in socialized leather/BDSM/kink from my teens. But I first got heavily involved in the clubs and organizations when I moved to Los Angeles from New York in 1980.

I attended a few Avatar Club Los Angeles meetings and then attended a play party they hosted. I wasn't known in Los Angeles yet as a player. I ended up topping a guy I met at the party itself. About an hour into the scene I realized I was being watched. I turned around and a small crowd had gathered. Afterwards, someone from the club came up to me and said, "Would you be interested in teaching some of us what you know?" My BDSM teaching path was born. I taught one class for them, then many others, ended up on their Board of Directors, and the rest is history.

When I first entered the scene, gay leathermen didn't really obsess about labels much. We mostly just generically referred to ourselves as top, versatile or bottom and only occasionally something else. I came out directly into BDSM as a top/Dom and stayed there for about 20 years. It wasn't until the early 90s that I began to slowly (very slowly) explore being a switch (versatile), at least in terms of BDSM. Sexually I was always sort of versatile, meaning that on rare occasions I would bottom, but when it came to BDSM I only topped.

It's a funny story how I very publicly came out as starting to explore being a switch. My ex, Guy Baldwin, and I were at a play party, in Portland. It was in a huge dungeon with perhaps 150-200 people in it. I had just topped Guy in a hot scene and we were taking a break. At that point, our relationship was beginning to wind down, yet we were still extremely close. We both decided to walk around the dungeon separately to see what other trouble we might want to get into. About a half hour later we came together again and I recall Guy saying, "You're the most interesting guy here, do you want to get whipped?" For some reason I said yes. Guy tied me up and flogged me. At one point dozens of people were watching, with many expressing surprise I was bottoming and that Guy was topping me. I guess I figured if you're going to come out as a switch, you might as well do it big.

When you first enter the scene, especially the organized scene, you believe deeply that your BDSM identity, preferred kinks and relationship dynamics are set in stone. You truly believe, "This is how I am and this is how I'll always be." Then the reality sets in that the only constant is change, and that applies as much to people and BDSM as it does to everything else.

Today I identify as a switch, but increasingly I am eschewing labels. Sometimes I'm in high Dom mode. Other times I might feel more submissive. Most of the time I'm an opportunist and I say, "Show me the person and I'll tell you what's possible."

I've gone from a staunch top and Dom to an occasional switch who openly seeks out all types of power dynamics and activities in my BDSM. I've gone from having a few specific, but simple, BDSM techniques in my toolkit, to be being considered by many to be one of the most technically proficient BDSM players in the world, and now to reeling my toolkit back to the few types of activities that seem to really satisfy me most. I've gone from reveling in the labels placed on me and caring what people think of me to not really embracing labels much and not caring so much what others think.

I have no desire to be bonded to anyone long-term from a bottom or submissive standpoint. That might change, but my desire to be the Dom in BDSM has been solid and consistent. I currently have two men collared. My BDSM takes place outside of my primary relationship. Both of my slaves also have their own primary partners. They live on their own apart from me (I live with my two primary partners).

I met my life-partner nearly 25 years ago. He started out as my slave, but after about three years our relationship morphed into a more traditional structure. He and I met our other partner nearly 20 years ago.

The three of us have been cohabitating ever since and consider ourselves a triad.

Balancing my BDSM and kink needs with my triad can be challenging. One issue has arisen that's been problematic for one of my triad partners and we continue to wrestle with it. I need very close bonding to those with whom I have power-based relationships, and power-based relationships are extremely important to me and my erotic fulfillment. As Joseph Bean [*BDSM author, former Executive Director of the Leather Archives & Museum*] once pointed out in Rule 5 of his wonderful *10 Rules of SM*, "If you're not in love, don't do the scene." Of course, I see love as a many-faceted thing and there is an endless array of permutations of love, but some form of actual love is vital for me when in a power-based relationship. I'm not sure how it will be resolved because to turn my back on power-based relationships is to turn my back on the very core of my kink needs.

A person can be taught the basics of BDSM culture, safety and technique rather easily and quickly. Yet, the non-stop abundance of BDSM classes often gives both newcomers and experienced players alike the impression that they need to continually attend a bevy of classes in order to be an "approved" BDSM player. I think that's a dangerous message to send, even if it's sent unintentionally. And I do know some who send the message intentionally. People who actually believe all BDSM players should always be attending additional BDSM classes.

We're the most overeducated subculture around. We worship at the altar of education and I think in many ways it might be harming us more than helping us. We've gotten lazy with our education. We rarely vet the instructors well. We rarely give any deep thought to an appropriate curriculum progression. We think that giving more classes is a sign of an event or group's success, even if some classes were of dubious quality. True success would be to offer fewer classes but of higher quality. We also err on the side of classroom-style instruction with students watching and listening rather than hands-on, experiential learning. I believe that when it comes to technique BDSM instructions, hands-on is really the only way to go if you really want to create effective learning situations.

The biggest challenge in BDSM relationships is facing the realities of change. Changes in relationship structures. Changes in the levels of erotic need and the types of erotic needs. Changes that come with aging or illness. Changes in power direction flows. Nothing is constant except change, and BDSM is no exception. We change and the scene around us changes daily. We can't ignore that reality. We have to adapt and change with it.

One of the greatest minds of the BDSM scene and a friend, Tony DeBlase [aka "Fledermaus," creator of the Leather Pride Flag] hammered home to me repeatedly that we must never become slaves to technique. We must never elevate technique to a place where it trumps the internal connections and visceral erotic joy that good BDSM brings about. To do so does, in my opinion, demean BDSM and relegate it to nothing more than a bit of technical acumen rather than the mechanism by which people intimately connect.

*Lady Elaina

Beginning on the bottom, Elaina has evolved into a femdom, club founder and leader who focuses on teaching tolerance and preventing interpersonal abuse.

I want to thank you for including me, as Slave V (my nom de plume), in the first book. I am actually known as Lady Elaina. I was 38 years old at the time I was interviewed, so I'm 61 now. I had just opened my small business, Samco, manufacturer of SceneWear® Originals. I started it while looking for another position in International Institutional Finance on Wall Street, my actual profession.

In almost every job I had, I was the first woman ever to hold that position. I like to break through barriers, I guess, and I feel naturally drawn to lead. And just because something has always been the purview of men, I don't allow that to deter me from going after it, if I want it. In fact, I found a new position during the time of your interviews, and returned to my career in New York City, while continuing to run Samco on the side. I retired from that powerful and exciting career too early, due to a catastrophic car accident. I have been able to achieve partial recovery, but remain disabled as far as prolonged walking and standing. Thankfully, I have disability insurance until I am 65.

Now that I am retired from my career on Wall Street, I've had more time for Samco, and it's grown nicely. I design our clothing and leather, do all procurement, leather making, etc. I can be "out" without worry, so everyone knows me as Lady Elaina, Master of the Unicorn Household, at Unicorn Keep. (I selected that name after someone told me that the M/s Switch is a mythological creature, like the Unicorn, LOL.)

I am not sure that I had many expectations from BDSM other than blockbuster orgasms! Not surprisingly, I had the young woman's dream of finding a wonderful Master and making a life together. But I chose poorly with a few men, and the one man I chose well died of brain cancer early in my journey. That has been the biggest disappointment. I was not able to make a successful life with a mentally healthy, loving Dominant Man.

The relationship I described in the original book turned out to be the kind of abusive nightmare that we try to educate people to avoid. I ignored the warnings I got from people who knew him, as women tend to do when they are not thinking with the right part of their anatomy. "He won't do that to me," I thought. Well, yup... he did. He ruptured a disk in my neck and cleaned me out financially. I had to get rescued by scene friends. The extensive financial, physical and psychological damage from that relationship took me over four years to emerge from. Plus he stalked me for 10 years, showing up at my vendor booths at out-of-state events. Slave Rob (my hunky D/s slave who has been with me 18 years now, and lives in the New York City house), would chase him away. I tried to warn his new girlfriend, who came with him once, and she said (you guessed it), "He won't do that to me."

Through groups I founded in New Jersey, I've tried to share knowledge, but also to show how much better things can be when done from a place of knowledge and love. It's largely about intent. If it comes from a place of love, it is very unlikely to go wrong. Unfortunately, sometimes abuse is consensual and comes from low self-esteem. Those who are abused often cannot extract themselves, or even see it sometimes, as I learned the hard way. Sadly, those who need it most are the ones who most resist it. Still, we have to promote education about it. Should one play into a sub's low self-esteem? Or a master's egoistic self-aggrandizement? Is it healthy for slaves to address themselves in the third person as objects or does it do self-harm? Just because someone will consent to something, does that mean it's okay to do it? Abuse is not the same as feeding a masochist in a loving way.

I am no longer as ruled by my gonads, but yes, it is, when it comes to BDSM I do love rope. Now that I am older, I mostly end up tying up other people. Most men like to tie up young ladies, not old ones. Also, older bodies cannot take as much stress. Mine certainly can't after all the surgeries. I do still dream about receiving it, the desire hasn't gone away, at least not yet. Of course, with an ongoing lack of positive rein-forcement, in time, I expect that I will lose interest in doing it altogether. I do get offers for sex, of course, but not from the right men. And un-fortunately, I need to be in a relationship for the play to produce the sort of effect I crave. It is still possible I could feel submission to a man, but he would have to be very special and spiritually enlightened. There is a small part of me that still hopes for it, but it gets smaller with the passage of time and the increase in my disability.

I became bored with BDSM in the late 90's, after about 18 years of do-ing it, the last 10 years of which were in the public scene. I found that the submission of only the body began to get old. The same old stuff, different day. I began to ask, "...is that all there is?" and considered leav-ing it all behind. Instead, I moved on to a far more interesting playing field for me, called M/s [ed. Master/slave]. It entails the surrender of the mind, and the responsibility for accepting that surrender, with all its implications. I have been a Master for about 10 years now and active in the M/s community. In fact, I presented at the M/s Conference (2014), in Washington, DC, on Financial Planning for M/s Households. Cross that one off my bucket list!

When I finally ventured out into BDSM again after my abusive relation-ship, I followed the advice of that friend, who said, "You were the Auc-tioneer at Paddles, you know how to act dominant, so go out as a Domme. Go to Jersey where they don't really know you; no one will be the wiser." So I did just that because, as I said, "If I am in charge, at least no one gets hurt."

I was not submissive again for 11 years. I then had a D/s Master, starting in 2003, for about 3½ years, while also having a collared M/s slave, a D/s slave, and a BDSM sub. (A condition of accepting the Master into my life was that I was permitted to keep my obligations to my slaves/sub, and he consented.) It was easy at first, as the Master was in Philadelphia and the slaves/sub were in New York City. However, when I moved mostly to the Philadelphia area, many of the less enlightened people could not accept that I was an M/s Switch. The M/s community continues to reject M/s Switches as a valid identity, and will even go as far as to shun them. I hold an annual luncheon for switches at the M/s Conference, and some folks don't attend the lunch for fear of the repercussions of being seen there.

The scene opened my eyes about human power dynamics at a level that most regular folks probably don't consider. My advice pertains to everyone: watch out for the unhealthy people who hide among us.... they are numerous and often tell a good story. Sometimes they are obviously angry people, and sometimes they are slick like a snake. Listen when people warn you that someone has a bad reputation. Don't jump into the lifestyle with so much trust that people hurt you. Take your time, if it is any good, it can wait a minute. Just because it is on the Internet, doesn't mean that Master Moron has an opinion you should respect. Listen to respected leaders, there is a reason they are considered leaders! And get many different opinions about *everything*.

Lastly, and most of all, whether you are the top or the bottom, remember what Guy Baldwin said in his book, *SlaveCraft*: "protect the property."

slave matt

A long-time BDSM player with a public reputation to protect, in private matt is submissive to his dominant wife.

I knew as a child that BDSM was exciting. I didn't put it together, though, until college. Even when I was finally able to put a name to my desires, I still felt fearful about acting on them. I finished college, did three years of grad school, and soon after married at age 27. The marriage was friendly but passionless and my libido mostly went into suspended animation. My first wife, or maybe that whole first marriage, convinced me that I had little to no libido.

Then in 1984 I bought a modem, signed up for CompuServe, and, recalling old interests, wandered into a BDSM/leather chatroom. I got pretty active, made a few friends, but never had the nerve to tell my wife about my growing interests, much less to consummate my perverse longings. (Though I did make one visit to a pro dominatrix in the late 1990s.)

My second marriage has shown me very much otherwise about my libido, and my BDSM lusts are a good part of that. It wasn't until I fell in love with the woman who is now my second wife – and Mistress – that I really opened up. Early in our relationship (as it was breaking up my first marriage, not coincidentally) I told her all about my unusual desires. She was open to them, though she wasn't there yet. I did ultimately manage to seduce her into this lifestyle, however, and to draw out her inner sadist, and now we're in a heavily, though not entirely, BDSM relationship.

Over time, I discovered that one of the hardest things about submission for me was learning to give up my ego, at least temporarily. It's taken us a long time to get to the point where severe teasing and humiliation excite me, but now we're there. The daily life angle of BDSM in a marriage is complicated. I think we both want more of a kinky power dynamic in the day-to-day, but then I resist, or we forget/get distracted. But there is always a power buzz going, especially if I'm locked up in a cock cage. When I'm locked, I always think I should be submissive even if I'm not always.

I'm madly in love with my wife. All this perverse/poly stuff makes us love each other more. I'm 62 now but if I could talk to myself as a young man, I'd say, "Go for it, wanker. Don't be so inhibited." Now I want to evangelize to adults. So many of our friends are in sexless or near-sexless marriages or relationships. Some of it is the stifling hand of monogamy. Open up!

*Eve Howard

A vibrant and unique presence in the BDSM world, Eve has been sharing her love of spanking for three decades while helping millions of others find their fetish joy.

I was 37 when I was first interviewed and I'm 60 today. I'm married to Tony, my partner of 28 years and we live in Las Vegas. Our long-time partner in Shadow Lane, Butch Simms, lives next door. Being as entrenched in the scene as I am, the label "lifestyle" fits me in the literal sense. Still, while living it 24/7 is something dreamers dream of doing, it isn't very practical. Even the most idealistic purists are not in the mood to play 24/7.

In 1991, my first Shadow Lane book was just about to come out in paperback and our 14th video had just been released. Over the last 23 years, I've continued writing Shadow Lane novels and volume twelve will be printed this year. Shadow Lane has also published numerous spanking magazines and personal ads publications. We have been helping spanking people make romantic and play connections for over twenty-five years. We've also helped people who couldn't find fruitful spanking interactions on their own to connect with professional spankers and spankees. We continue to be active in all of these activities.

My transitional step into the spanking world was becoming a freelance editor for Lyndon Publications, where I took over a magazine they had just started up called *Spank Hard* in the middle 1980's. I moved from the cut and dried world of adult publications to the passionately obsessed niche fetish industry. Once I began writing columns, I heard from collectors, film historians, compulsive novel searchers. I related to them all because I'd been similarly obsessive in my own search for spanking references my entire life. Everyone wrote me but women. Women didn't go into adult bookstores looking for spanking magazines at that time because there weren't any worth finding. But they did read *Cosmo* and *Penthouse Variations* and I later found them there through tiny classified ads once I had my own videos and publications to sell. The female-friendliness of Shadow Lane publications, videos and personal ads, brought us female customers, female party guests and also female models drawn directly from the scene.

It was Ed Lee who wrote me a personal ad that drew a reply from Tony. Tony and I knew immediately that we were meant for each other. The first time we met, Tony was amazed that I was the real Lizzie Bennett (my pen name at *Spank Hard*), whose columns he had been reading for about a year. I was delighted to meet a young, good looking, confident top who was single and lived fifteen minutes away from me. It was just good all the way around. Almost as soon as we became a couple, we became a production team.

If it hadn't been for Ed Lee, there never would have been a Shadow Lane. He created a company that became the backbone of the American scene in the 1980's, producing an enormous library of authentic spanking videos that were distinctly American in flavor at a time when English caning videos were pretty much the only corporal punishment material on the market. No one in the world ever did more to define, expand, advance and celebrate the spanking scene. And because he put so much out there that was good and real, his products had the effect of reassuring thousands of enthusiasts that they were not alone, not crazy and not wrong to be obsessed with spanking. Ed Lee passed away on January 6, 2013, at the age of 73. There will never be another like him and he will be missed as no other, especially by me.

The spanking scene has furnished me with a more colorful and exhilarating social life than I could have ever enjoyed in the vanilla world. I'm shy, but in the scene, I can express myself without reserve. Many spanking enthusiasts have confided to me that like myself, in the world of vanilla society, they are painfully bashful and never know what to say at a party to strangers. In the spanking world, we have our own culture, our own language, and our own common experiences to bind us together from the moment we meet.

The spanking scene also proves the point so aptly made by Hunter S. Thompson, that, "When the going gets weird, the weird turn pro." I'm probably one of the better examples of that. When I worked in the

mainstream porn industry, no one ever noticed me. With my conservative appearance and eyeglasses, my place was behind the typewriter,
turning out the hot scenarios, but never being in them. Whereas, the
first thing the first spanking producer I met wanted to do with me was
spank me on video. Spanking people just don't mind nerdy girls or guys.
It kind of goes with the territory. Not to say there aren't super cool and
even super beautiful people into spanking too. But they don't necessarily have any more fun in the scene than ordinary folks or even geeky
ones.

I have lived my spanking fantasies to the full and beyond. I feel sorry for
straight people. Their realm of experience seems limited in comparison
to the possibilities offered by the fetish world.

How many vanillas do you know who just *play* with each other? What
would they even do to call it play? Dribble food items into each other's
mouths? Erotic massage? Slow strip teases? You could die of boredom
waiting for a straight person to come up with something new and interesting as a preface to or substitute for sex.

Action fetishes like spanking, bondage, femdom worship, cross dressing,
etc., when enacted with like-minded play partners, are the apotheosis of
foreplay. Playing is a leisurely pastime, full of ritual and protocol,
providing a slow erotic build-up of tension and excitement. Playing is
dynamic sensory stimulation that melds imagination with physicality,
often resulting in transcendently ecstatic experiences, such as floating
in "sub space" or climaxing through spanking alone. Whether fetish play
results in actual sex or not, it can still be engaging, amusing, arousing
and satisfying.

Aldous Huxley said, "The only really completely consistent people are
dead." When I first came out I just didn't think any role but spankee
would ever suit me. There are plenty of male tops to go around for
those women who only wish to receive. But the very first session I ever
did as a pro sub, the client turned out to be a switch. I did not see that
coming. I went with it and soon found out that switchable guys exist in
numbers too big to ignore. Flexibility turned out to be a better match
for me, especially as I get older. I can and do still sub, but not in the
random, thrill-seeking style I formerly embraced. I'm naturally bossy
and being a disciplinarian lets me have fun with that, ideally while
providing a turn-on to someone else.

Almost as soon as I began playing as a top I noticed a difference in my own emotions about meeting a stranger for a scene. Whenever I was going to get spanked by someone for the first time, I would feel tense, uneasy and full of trepidation. Sometimes the stress would give me a migraine. I had to prepare mentally and half the time I dreaded the encounter for one reason or another, but mainly for fear of severe pain. I'm into spanking but I'm not a masochist.

On the other hand, when going out to top a stranger for the first time, I didn't need mental prep time. I felt content and carefree, and the idea of spanking, paddling, strapping or caning a stranger gave me zero stress. As long as I have enough time to pack my oversized artist's portfolio full of leather and wood, my head is there.

The spanking scene has extended my youth as well as that of most of my spanking girlfriends. In fact, it seems to me that the scene is a lot friendlier to mature women than the straight world. I remember as a teen in the late 1960's, reading of Monique Von Cleef, the famous Dutch mistress who wrote her memoirs. I was both appalled and fascinated by the fact that she was still sessioning in her seventies. It didn't seem possible yet now I'm topping in spanking videos myself. I know other ladies my age in the scene who are confident enough in their gym-toned glutes to still sub on camera and display their 1950's vintage realness as spankees. And their videos sell! Men get a similar break because daddies can come in all ages.

While the scene will always be about playing and sexual excitement, it offers so much more, including opportunities for lifelong friendships with people who share the fetish. I see spanking as a hobby as much as a sexual preoccupation. It encourages reading, writing, film history, photography, art, costume design and many other forms of creative self-expression as people search for new ways to live out their fantasies.

Nigel Cross

Nigel Cross is the nom-de-plume of a long-time male sub-missive. He writes femdom fiction and novels under this name.

It wasn't until I was in the U.S. Military that I actually started acting on my BDSM desires. After my experiences as a cadet, I was stationed at Presidio of San Francisco and my girlfriend at the time was an enlisted woman and fellow Korean language student stationed there with me. She knew a lot about San Francisco and started taking me to different downtown clubs that catered to a BDSM clientele. This was at a time when the BDSM scene was really underground, so finding these places meant being guided there by someone already in that community. She often introduced me as her submissive, and for the most part, people accepted me as that. Our relationship felt more vanilla than BDSM, even though she was very controlling and made most of the decisions when the two of us were together.

When I got out of the service, I really started to explore my submissive side as a lifestyle. I met two women who were both well-recognized professional dominants who were known nationwide (although I didn't know that at the time as I was still really new to the ins and outs of this industry). For the two weeks they were in town, they offered me the opportunity to be their personal slave, basically taking care of their every need while they were in town. I jumped at the chance. This meant driving them everywhere, escorting them to all sorts of different events, dressing them constantly, and serving as a personal servant for any whim they might have at any moment (and they had a lot of whims).

It was also the first time I was used for sex by a woman who tied me up and had her way with me. Strangely enough, it involved no money whatsoever (I guess I got lucky I wasn't first discovered by financial dommes instead of them). Those two weeks went by in a blur and remain that way in my memory today. When they returned home to Pennsylvania, they offered to make me their permanent slave if I decided to move there, but sadly, I was too stupid at the time to realize how great an opportunity they were offering me.

A few years later, I became the personal slave of a well-known professional dominant in San Francisco who ran a BDSM business out of her mansion of a home. I was her slave for several years before she left the business and didn't renew our yearly contract. I decided to avoid any further BDSM relationships but less than a month later I met a woman from Hong Kong, who I started dating with all intentions of remaining in a vanilla relationship. But by this time, I was a well-recognized submissive from the early days of the Internet, so it took very little effort for her to discover that I was well-known and had published lots of writing about submission.

Out of the blue she said, "Now I finally understand why you're the way you are," and then she vowed to become my new owner. That lasted a number of years until she discovered the pro domination world, became a pro domme and pretty much left me behind to pursue her new lifestyle. She's actually quite well-known today as a professional dominant.

I can honestly say it was a common pattern that a vanilla woman dated me, discovered I was a submissive, decided to be dominant, discovered the pro domination industry and then left me for that new life. It happened so many times I thought it was a cosmic joke.

When I first started out as a submissive, I spent a lot of time discussing the lifestyle with people who were exploring this aspect of themselves as well. It was at the dawn of the Internet, when submissives were basically expected to be silent and only observe. A female submissive friend of mine and I created an organization called The Submissive Treehouse. It helped to usher in a more accommodating atmosphere for those who were once afraid to identify as BDSMers. Over the years, I became an officer in a number of BDSM and femdom organizations with the sole purpose of helping others connect in a world that can act very negative towards our lifestyle. I've also written a number of novels about femdom relationships.

For me, developing BDSM relationships has always been relatively easy. I think it's because I'm honest about what I am. There are a lot of falsehoods in this Community that keep people from achieving the relationships they want, such as a submissive who pretends to be something he or she might not be because he or she wants to attract a certain dominant, dominants who realize that the cadre of submissives willing to offer what they want are actually limited, and people who don't even know what they want but are willing to do anything to appeal to other people long enough to try to figure out what it is they might have wanted in the first place.

The hardest thing for me was accepting myself as a submissive. I live in a male dominant world, a patriarchy of crappy ideals. I went to West Point where I was taught to be a leader (even in my completely fucked up way) and where people assumed I was a leader. And in certain contexts, I've had to assume that identity. But femdom relationships are the only ones that have ever worked for me. After 30 years in the lifestyle, I've never stopped being submissive. I have an owner I serve to this day.

Some people have assumed because it's some kind of reaction to my straight life. It isn't. It's because I'm most comfortable in this role. I feel wonderful when I'm doing something for a woman I care about. When I see her smile and acknowledge that I was important to her because of my submissive acts, I'm at the top of my world. When I am needed by her, desired by her (not just sexually but just in a general sense of being), and appreciated by her, I can't imagine another place I would rather be. The accoutrements of our lifestyle are great and can be great turn-ons, but they pale in magnitude to the wondrous revelation you receive when she smiles and shows how pleased she is with just being in the same room as you, and you know you exist as something that only makes her life that much better.

Lolita Wolf

An historic figure in the national BDSM/leather scene, aka "Leather Yenta," Lolita is one of the Scene's most knowledgeable experts in all aspects of safe play.

The biggest lesson I've learned over the years is that BDSM is never what I think it's going to be. It is always different. And it always changes. For example, what interested me 30 years ago is different from what I wanted 10 years ago, which is different from what I want today. A lot of what happens depends on the people I'm with. I've learned not to try and push people into the roles that I want them to play with me, but rather to find the relationship that works well for us both as we are. By applying that philosophy, it seems that whatever I need comes my way.

These days, I'm much more top-leaning and, as a bottom, I'm really a do-me queen. I don't have as much patience doing things outside my specific preferences because I'm older now, and pretty much want what I want when I want it. I'll still bottom casually sometimes, but it has to be something I really want to do. I bottomed to someone recently who was kind of new to all this, and it was so boring. I felt like, "Oh crap, okay, I'll take it for the team, but meh." LOL

My all-time best BDSM relationship is the one I have now. He's my best friend. We don't pressure each other, we recognize we each have baggage, and we don't have huge, unrealistic expectations of each other. You know how you have a close friend who you're always there for when they need you, and they are always there for you when you need them? That's the foundation for my love relationship with my partner. We've been doing this for nine years.

My other BDSM relationships were good, each one had some great qualities, but they have ended, and they ended for their own reasons. I'm older and smarter now, and I have different priorities today than in the past. I'm a much better communicator too.

I see a lot of people in relationships where people aren't really whole. I am a whole person whether or not I'm in a relationship. I keep a little distance. I am very independent. I see a lot of people being very clingy and needy in their relationships. They'll say, "This person completes me." I feel I am already a complete person. A relationship isn't what defines my happiness, I define it. I don't sit around waiting for the phone to ring. I'm busy with work, and friends, and life. Most importantly, I am my own person. That means I have the strength and maturity to allow the person I'm involved with to be their own person too, without trying to manipulate them into living up to a fantasy ideal.

I am still poly, and have other things going on, and so does he. That makes it even better for me. Before I found the BDSM scene, whenever I was in a relationship, I felt that life was passing me by because I was stuck in a relationship. But then whenever I wasn't in a relationship, I felt bad because I missed the intimacy of a relationship. What a mess. When I got into the scene, I realized, wow, I could have both! Wow, I can eat my cake and have it too! Wow!

I teach poly classes now. For me, it would be a challenge not to be poly. It gives me the freedom to be anything I want to be. What's so fabulous and unique about my guy is that he accepts all those things that I am and even thinks that it's hot. I think that about him too! At first, he had another partner who was very jealous, so he felt like he had to sneak around to be with me. So it took a while for him to realize that he didn't have to lie to me as he did to his ex. It makes me really happy to hear all his stories. They're fun to listen to, they bring us closer, and the honesty makes me feel very secure with him.

I haven't stopped evolving. I am still open to change. I think a lot of people are married to their roles. They're not being authentic. I know someone who got deeply involved in the M/s community after being a switch like me. He said, "But I really miss bottoming." So I said, "Well? So do it." And he said, "Oh, no, I can't because I'm a master."

So sometimes people are not true to themselves because they get trapped in a role. Or there are those who try to be something they're not because they believe it's what their partners expect of them. "OMG, now I have to be this and do that, and I know there are things I'm not allowed to do because I'm a master and masters don't do that." That's all bullshit.

Some people simply cannot separate fantasy from reality. They start believing things that just aren't real. For example, they will imagine that if they signed a BDSM contract it means you can't back out of it. I've talked to plenty of people who say they want to stick out a bad relationship because they are afraid of failing at it. I want to tell them that it isn't their failure when their partner can't or won't give them what they need emotionally. At that point, you have to walk away. You see similar things in vanilla relationships, but some situations are unique to BDSM. So, for us, keeping your feet on the ground, and knowing where fantasy ends and reality begins is not just important, it is fundamental to informed consent.

BDSMers 50+

Stephanie Locke

Legendary dominatrix, Stephanie is internationally renowned for her exceptional skills, commitment to BDSM, and contributions to popularizing the Mistress/slave lifestyle.

After reading a story about a woman who had slaves, I started dreaming and plotting, at age 9, how to become one of the greatest Mistresses in the world. I just knew it was my future. We moved around a lot in my childhood, so I bided my time, figuring that we'd eventually move to a city where I could find posh SM clubs like the one in the book and find my own slaves.

When I was 16, my family was transferred to a military base in Germany. Until then I'd been dressing the way my mother wanted me to, in very lady-like outfits, which I didn't care for. But at the base, I met a group of guys who agreed to get me a pair of jeans. It took all four of them to get me into those super tight jeans, and from then on, my style changed. One of the guys turned out to be a fetishist. He asked if he could shave my legs. I was thinking, "OMG, OMG, he's a slave," though I didn't say it out loud. Afterwards, we went out to the pool where he had arranged a silver plate for me filled with hundreds of dollars.

At 17, I left home because I wasn't getting along with my mother. I ended up in Hollywood, on Santa Monica Boulevard. I lived and worked and made friends with gay hustlers, who were very protective and kind to me. I approached a woman I trusted and asked her, "Are there any dungeons here?" She was shocked to hear me ask about SM. I explained that I wanted to do this since I was nine. Reluctantly, she told me about one she knew, so I went there right away.

After thinking up some brilliant lies to tell about my age because I was still only 17, I met the owner of the dungeon. He immediately took to me. He told me he'd invented someone exactly like me before we even met. I fit his ideal perfectly, including my eyeglasses and height (5'9"). He saw great potential in me, and predicted that I would be one of the most famous Mistresses the world had ever known. He had a few important pieces of advice for me. For one, he insisted that I keep both a first and last name professionally, and not allow myself to be known just by a first name. He felt it added credibility. Second, he said I never should abandon the glasses. He said they would be like a style signature for me, and he was right, they did.

I worked there about 9 months but finally came to the depressed realization that I was simply too young. I was not ready. I wept over it and then I quit. I drifted and went to school and wandered and moved back in with my parents. One night, my father confronted me about what I was doing with my life. I told him, "Daddy, I want to be the greatest Mistress in the world." He said, "I hope not." Of course, it was too late by then. My mind was made up. I knew I belonged in that world.

In 1982, I called the Padded Cell, a small dungeon that an old friend once told me about. The owner wanted to hire me right away, on one condition: that I train as a submissive for a year. I told him there was no way. He started negotiating down to 6 months but I still could not imagine being submissive. Finally, he said, okay one month and I said okay. But from the first day I did sessions, I clearly had the makings of a dominant. Most of my sessions that first day were with submissives, and none of them even realized I was inexperienced. That was exhilarating. I never looked back after that.

By 21, I was able to open my own SM venue, called Club O, after *Story of O*. With my husband at the time, I'd already begun crafting my image as a dominatrix – choosing the best lingerie and the finest rubber and the softest leathers, and building up wardrobes. I have kept each and every toy, and every single garment, down to the garter belts, from my entire career. It's all stored now. It's an amazing collection I hope to donate one day to a costume archive or museum.

The 1980s were filled with paranoia and insecurities and police harassment, but the 1990s were great years for me professionally. The majority of our clients in the 1990s were from the top echelons of society – surgeons, movie directors, and some of the richest, smartest men in the world. There was a clutch of us, seven femdoms, in different cities around the world, and we more or less traded this group of men back and forth, depending on where the men were traveling. It was an amazing sorority of women, and we were very good to each other.

A number of challenges face professional femdoms. Not only do you need all the wardrobe and shoes and toys, but you need the attitude and self-confidence. Then you have to draw lines between your professional life and your private one. When it comes to really intimate things, like piercing, strap-ons, or enemas, I will not do them for money. I only do them in an intimate personal relationship.

When you're dominant your courtship rituals are different too. It's difficult to admit to emotions, and the last thing you want to do is be perceived as submissive on any level. It's tough to let your inner soft girl out. It's hard to know when it's safe to let her out. How do you trust a man when you know women are so often betrayed by men?

So how do you express your feelings? Well, for example, how do I convey to him that I care about his pleasure? I'll tell him, "Tonight, my corset is cinched to 19 inches, I've selected lingerie from the best boutique in Europe, I'm wearing insanely expensive heels, and I've set aside the most exquisite whip. See? I went to all that effort just for you." And how do I say I love you? I put him in a hood, and I put him in a straitjacket, I tie him down, and then maybe I'll suck his cock. That's how I say I love you.

In my 30s, it was very hard to say things like "I love you," "I care," or "I need." I selected only brilliant men because they needed more sophisticated sexuality that required more sophisticated dialogues. I needed to be able to talk to a man, not just about sex and SM, but a wide range of subjects, whether it is architecture or Ancient Roman history. But when one of them would ask to get more serious or propose marriage, I wouldn't talk to him again. It was over immediately. I didn't want to change my life for a man. I knew that when I sat down to dinner with so-called normal people, communication was always awkward. I belonged among that rare breed of women who wanted to dominate people and be a Mistress with slaves. I would never fit into suburbia.

Men are sluts. I mean, most men mean well but they can't help themselves. LOL. Once upon a time, maybe in the 1950s and 1960s, men were more honorable, and they did come home and treasure their wives. But we now live in what I call the post-Hallmark world. People still play the roles in public – they buy flowers and a Hallmark card that says I love you, but on the side they're watching porn, patting women on the head and pretending everything's fine.

My advice to men is that while it's important to let go and dive deeply into SM, in the end you do best to pick one woman and stick with her, and then let your kinks blossom with her. You honor her, whether she is your dominant or your submissive. You lavish her with luxuries and attentions. You make her the only important one in your life.

Meanwhile, if you've played for 15 years and you've played with lots of other partners, and it's starting to feel hollow, or you find yourself saying, "I love you," for the 15th time or you're wearing your 10th owner's collar, it's time to take a year off and work on your shit!

A lot of men have very unrealistic expectations. When they discover submission they suddenly believe they should be sexually aroused all the time. "Will you do me now? Will it happen now?" They start constantly craving the thrill. Sure, you can spank or whip someone a few times a day, but when men expect you to be in full dom mode 24/7, it's both exhausting and impractical. When they are expecting that every day is a scene, an enema, a bondage session, with dressing up, it really just wears the woman out.

If you try to live as a slave 24/7, holding to this fantasy of being in unending submission while she constantly dominates you, she will simply start to hate you at a certain point. If you think you don't deserve to sleep with a woman because you're too submissive, where does that leave her? You have to think back to before you discovered SM. You probably only had sex a couple or few times a week. Whatever was your normal then should be your normal in SM, unless both of you mutually want more.

I've been partnered with a woman for thirteen years, though we're currently in a state of change. I no longer keep a dungeon. When my elderly mother moved to Los Angeles two years ago, I needed to make room for her to stay with me, so I packed everything away. But I've never stopped being a Mistress. From January 1982 to right now in 2015, I have always had slaves in my life. As I said, I've kept every piece of equipment I've ever used. BDSM still matters that much to me in my life. Thirty-five years later and every single time I do it, something new happens. I call it the Bondage Miracle. I confess that after all the different things I've explored, bondage is still my favorite. It always feels new, every single time. I love BDSM and I always will.

*Kiri Kelly

Today a private player, Kiri was a popular young beauty who appeared in numerous spanking videos and fetish magazine shoots in the 1990s.

I was 33 when I was first interviewed. Today, I'm 55. I have my own business as a real estate photographer in Florida. My journey was definitely not what I expected... I had no idea it would take so long and that I would be in my 50's before I finally found what I had been searching for!

BDSM in general brought a world of exciting experiences to me that I feel privileged to have had and make me feel that I truly LIVED my life and did not merely exist. Unfortunately, it was a significant factor in the demise of my first two marriages. My husbands would go through the motions, but their lack of interest was obvious and I could tell that their heart wasn't in it. As a result, my desires weren't satisfied and I found myself miserable. I was able to part as friends with both men, but after the failure of my second marriage, I realized that I would never be truly happy without BDSM as a facet of my relationship and set out on a journey to find the Dominant gentleman of my dreams.

I will always treasure my years as Kiri Kelly and my fetish model/actress career. It gave me the gift of meeting like-minded friends and mentors in the BDSM world. I had some invaluable experiences that I will always cherish in memory. For the first time in my life, I had a feeling of normality and the feeling that I'd found my home. Still, though I had achieved a certain amount of fame as Kiri Kelly, I was also aware that the videos and magazines that I was in were Adult Stores. After being in *Different Loving*, I was proud to be able to say that I was interviewed in a book that could be found at any local bookstore. It added what I would describe as a "legitimacy" to how I felt about my career.

Since retiring from my video career and moving to Florida to search for that one special person to share my life with, I have been fortunate to meet some dear friends, but they were vanilla friends and once again I found that there was a tremendous loneliness, knowing that I was the only kinky one there.

I would try to convey my frustrations to my girlfriends by explaining that the saying, "There are plenty of other fish in the sea," didn't apply to someone who was kinky. Not only do you need to find a general compatibility and chemistry, but finding someone who was also kinky narrowed the sea to a lake. And within the BDSM world, there are so many different fetishes and levels of play, that finding someone who was actually into the same kinks as you turned that lake into a puddle. Then add trying just "to bump into" someone who shares the same BDSM desires in the vanilla world makes it feel like the search is next to impossible.

I spent many years searching through personal ads and such, but rarely connected with anyone. I did enjoy a year as a collared slave to a wonderful gentleman, but found that where I had a wonderful love with my husbands, but no kinky satisfaction, I enjoyed a great kinky play life with him, but couldn't get my heart to fall in love.

It wasn't until meeting my current husband and Master that I had the chance to put the two together and finally enjoy a fun and satisfying kinky sex life with him while also being head over heels in love with him. Today, I'm part of a poly family, where I consider myself to have a husband and a wife. We had our Commitment Ceremony on 12/12/12 at a resort on Sanibel Island in front of my parents, their siblings, children and grandchildren, and a few of our dearest friends.

In our private life, our husband is the Master of our family, and my wife and I are his collared submissives. I have developed a dominant side with my wife as well and she considers me her Mistress. BDSM opened me up to new possibilities. I had always searched for a singular man to marry, but my involvement in the BDSM world introduced me to my husband and wife and the poly world, which I would never have considered before, and has led to the love of not just one but two people. My biggest disappointment is that I am not able to legally marry my husband and wife, while my biggest surprise would be ending up with a husband AND a wife. It took a while for them to convince me to give the poly lifestyle a try, but I can't imagine life without either of them now!

I can't speak strongly enough to the importance for me of being part of a community of other kinky folks. I felt like an alien from another planet when I was growing up because of my desires. Only being around vanilla people can make you feel weird or strange about yourself. In my head, I would try to remind myself that the vanilla people were the strange ones who would limit themselves to such narrow experiences. I would try to hang on to my pride by knowing that it was a positive that I enjoyed all the flavors and spices in the sexual realm. But it wasn't easy and often just made me feel lonely.

My biggest regret is that I didn't seek out the local BDSM community in Florida sooner. I wasted many lonely years searching in all the wrong places for the right person(s) for me. When I finally found local events and munches, they helped me to feel "myself" again and showed me a path to finally meet my husband and wife. I am extremely grateful for our friends in the BDSM community. They continue to reinforce a healthy attitude as well as provide a world of entertainment and fun!

*Baby Glenn

A private player who embraced his diaper fetish to cope with disability, Glenn uses a pseudonym to protect his true identity.

As I noted in my first interview in 1991, BDSM and Adult Baby fantasies have made Multiple Sclerosis more tolerable for me. It's certainly given me some insights others wouldn't have, but I am not sure how much different things would have been if I never got MS. Maybe I would have loathed wearing diapers, along with a bunch of other things about having MS that I loathe. But I'd still be kinky, one way or another.

My wife doesn't really participate much in my fetish. My favorite nurse's aide is long since gone, as is another nice one that I found here and who worked for me for a number of years. I can't say that the fetish itself has done a lot for me beyond providing me with some stress relief, unless you count an extensive knowledge of baby products useful for a childless man of 52.

Some of the nicest surprises over the years were when I had nurses who generously indulged my fetishes and treated me like a baby. Perhaps they did it in part because it kept me from being irritable, I suspect, particularly during more serious flare-ups of the disease. In the 1980s, I thought by this age I would either be dead or get so sick of them that I'd go to any length to avoid wearing diapers. So it's been a pleasant surprise that despite HAVING to wear them because of MS, I realized I'd still WANT to wear diapers every now and then even if I was cured.

I guess my biggest disappointment has turned out to be that I am WAY more kinky than my wife, or, at least, a lot more open about expressing my kinkiness. I now realize that a traditional Catholic school education is NOT a ticket to mental health. My wife has really struggled with it, while I have a talent for ignoring troublesome priests. I've also found that it's VERY difficult for me, as a natural submissive, to ask for, much less require or demand, ANYTHING having to do with sex. I need to be prompted by the other dominant person. I recognize that it is a self-defeating loop and it's very annoying to me that I haven't broken out of it.

In summary, I really have not seen much change or had a lot of experience with BDSM since our original interview. I do participate in Internet chats, so I have some outlet for my interests, and keep an eye on changes in the BDSM scene. Still, I am very disappointed that I was never able to connect with more people like me in real life and that I haven't been able to get my wife to show more interest in it.

*Laura Antoniou

Author of a popular BDSM novel series, editor, activist, and educator, Laura has been active in the Community since the 1980s.

I was 29 when I was first interviewed in 1991. I had just started writing and selling erotic fiction, and was editing collections as well, and hadn't even decided which name to use. At the time, I was working in the AIDS community, writing erotica and non-fiction on the side, and starting to edit anthologies. Now, I am a full time writer, teacher and speaker on alternative sex topics. I am 50 years old. I'm out, period, in the name I was given as a baby, all across the spectrum, including my gay male erotica. I've also been given some attention for my first mystery novel, set in the modern leather/kinky community.

I was in a short-term relationship back then and looking for more. Then, I spent some years single, playing the field. Then, I fell in love and got married – in 1998 – and then after that hooked up with another woman with whom I've had a DS relationship outside my marriage. So my situation today is pretty fucking sweet.

Back then, I might have called myself anything. Bisexual? Sometimes. Lesbian? Sure. But really, back then and now, I am primarily a sadomasochist, period. I have a strong preference in love/romantic attachment – to women – and therefore am more likely to say "lesbian" in circles where "sadomasochist" isn't an option, or would just confuse people. Sadomasochism colors my life every day. It remains – as it always has been – the way I achieve pleasure, even if it's just the thought that triggers orgasm.

Life is nothing but a string of surprises and our reactions to them. The first big thing that changed for me was my complete loss of interest in public play. Not that I was ever an exhibitionist, but it was such a major part of my early years, I imagined it always would be. Nope! Don't like it, can't be bothered.

Later on, I was surprised that my need for physical intensity shifted way, way down. But that could have been depression and/or the medications treating it. But now, off meds and not depressed, I find I am still not the same sort of seeker I used to be. Still damn pervy, though.

The big disappointments have mainly been about how ethically and socially screwy the organized kinky communities can be. Petty power plays in local organizations, theft from national ones, hidden bookkeeping, lying and bad faith, bad behavior, tolerance of abuse and abusers... I try not to feel surprised anymore, but I often still am.

Still, I remain committed to the idea that perverts can find balance and health in their lives by embracing their needs and desires, communicating them with honesty and clarity, and learning how to reconcile the fantasies of fiction, porn, imagination and "community expectations" with the lives they actually live.

Seeing how power works and doesn't in relationships where people discuss these things alerts me to just how badly it can wind up when we don't, whether or not we acknowledge we're kinky. The endless heterosexual advice columns, books, movies, systems – on how to manipulate each other – women leading men to commitment, men leading women to sex – have always been far more insulting and degrading to the alleged "sanctity of opposite sex relationships" than any gay couple getting matching rings could ever be.

By the time *Different Loving* came out, I'd realized the problem with having multiple identities meant I was pretending a lot, and it didn't feel good. If I could talk to myself back then, I'd say, ditch the closet entirely – except for the gay stuff because no one would have bought those stories if they knew I was a woman. (Oddly enough, gay romance and erotica is now a professional field inhabited by VAST numbers of women, most of them straight! Funny world.)

The closet is not worth it. I want to do what I like, I want to do it well and be known for it. So, if I'm gonna write SM fairy tales of action and adventure and owners and slaves, I want them well written and I want people to know where to come to get them signed.

If I was giving myself advice back then, I'd tell myself to be much clearer when negotiating and to stop trying to be someone I wasn't to get dates. I'd also assure myself that I was doing the right thing by sticking with safer sex. I'd also tell myself to buy stock in Amazon and Apple.

Karen Kalinowski

Known to her fans as Karen the Sex Lady, she has been a popular sex and BDSM mentor for over two decades. She also advocates for survivors of sexual abuse.

I am currently 50 years old. My partner is 56. I identify in the same manner as I did when I first came into the public scene: pansexual, switch, with more Domme tendencies. My partner identifies as heterosexual, switch, with more submissive tendencies. We have been in a monogamous relationship for 24 years. That doesn't mean that we don't find other people attractive, but so far, neither of us has had enough interest in acting on those desires. We both present as cisgendered, although we are fairly androgynous when it comes to many lived aspects of our daily lives (division of household chores, parenting, etc.).

We live our BDSM status 24/7. We don't have a lot of the external signs that some BDSM people consider necessary, like the collar or a St. Andrew cross in the living room, but there is a general understanding that when my foot is placed into his lap when we are on the sofa, that service is required. Similarly, service is rendered to one another in chores that we do for one another. It is understood that he will make tea but that I will make dinner. Much of what we do would fly under the flag as regular partnered interactions but it is in the acknowledgement of the service that makes it different. We use a lot of silent commands and hand signals. It is our own private way of communicating our wants and desires.

For about 10 years, I used a pseudonym when I wrote erotica and my sex and kink advice column. Our child was young at the time and I worried about how we might be perceived if I was "outed" as being kinky. I had heard about other parents who had received visits from child welfare agencies as a consequence of their sexual interests. The thought of losing custody of our child kept me from attending anything where our real names might be known. Only one half of the family (my side) knew about my working life because my in-laws were deeply religious. Living that way felt deeply inauthentic to me, particularly when I regularly counseled people to live their truth. My partner and I really started attending events openly about ten years ago. I conduct public education workshops while he supports me by doing my technical aspects and occasionally being my demo dolly.

The impact of BDSM on our relationship has been a positive surprise. I had no idea that our level of communication would deepen as much as it has. When we were younger, we spent a lot of time discussing expectations, likes/dislikes, needs, desires. That conversation has never stopped as our play has evolved. Certainly there are times when words are not necessary (because we are reading one another's body language) but neither of us had any idea that these discussions would bring us to a greater understanding of who we are as human beings.

We also couldn't have anticipated that our sex life would be so enriched by kink or that it would be this good well into our fifties. I think that's something that vanilla communities might not get. When disability/aging/illness impacted our sexual relationship from time to time over the years, kink was still there for us. There is so much that can be done with the mind, a look and simple touch that can fan the flames of desire and meet the needs of all involved parties.

I see two big challenges facing those who want to form successful BDSM relationships. The first one is in connecting with the right person. Yes, there are events, such as munches/sloshes/play parties/social networking for kinky folks but that doesn't take into account all the interesting vanilla-ish people you could be missing out on meeting in ALL other communities. Finding the right match, particularly in smaller, rural locations can be a challenge, not because there aren't kinky people but they are afraid of outing themselves as such.

A second big challenge is that the definition of kink varies from person-to-person. For some, wearing a blindfold is ultra kinky, whereas others define kinky as being suspended while forced to achieve orgasm multiple times. Finding partners who match or accept your sexual orientation and fall within the same range of activities can be challenging.

I also want to mention how freeing kink can be for survivors of sexual abuse. I am a survivor and I really feel as though BDSM has allowed me to reclaim my sexuality through fantasy and other acts that are not sexual. I have a number of clients who have been helped by the negotiation required in kink to create a consensual scene. Feeling as though they can contribute and sometimes control how the scene will play out has been deeply therapeutic for many of the abuse survivors I've known. Many of them have even re-visited their abuse and turned it into something positive that they explore regularly.

Guy deBrownsville

Guy is a widely-respected founder, member and organizer of groups for People of Color, and is on the board of directors of the Eulenspiegel Society.

I always identified as Dominant, and in my current relationship I identify as an Owner. To me there is a difference as far as direct responsibility and it took me a while to get to a place where I felt comfortable with that degree of control and responsibility. The woman that I am with made it very easy for me to accept that about myself because of how she responds to me and what she sees in me. I am grateful to her for that.

Like many, though I was in my 40's when I formally got involved in the scene in 2001, I was relatively idealistic, wide-eyed and bushy-tailed when I first arrived. I didn't know what I didn't know. My first relationship didn't work out because I relied upon the fact that my partner had more time in the scene than I and assumed that we were on the same wavelength. I had failed to communicate what I was looking for adequately and I didn't really ask what she wanted or find out if we defined familiar terms the same way. I confess it took me years to be as communicative about those important things as I needed to be.

In addition, I bought into the notion of one big happy "Community." One comparison I've heard and like to repeat is when someone says, "I love wine." The drunk in the street and the wine connoisseur both "love wine" but that doesn't make them a community. BDSM is the same way. I learned that just because we all engage in BDSM, it doesn't make us a community. Moreover, the same divisions that are found in the world at large exist in the BDSM world. There are racial, cultural, political, economic, gender and sexuality based divides, among others. It took me a little while to realize I wasn't stepping into a utopia.

What also surprised me was just how broad the scope of BDSM is. You can take one thing, like electric play for instance, and it can vary from TENS units and violet wands which are relatively low sensation devices, to electric cattle prods and stun guns which are entirely at the other end of the spectrum. This is another reason why real dialogue is essential. Also, there is the idea that BDSM does not automatically include SM or even sex for that matter. Some people just like service or hierarchical relationships. The varying interpretations of BDSM are both surprising and fascinating to me.

The biggest challenge in forming BDSM relationships may be summed up with one word: trust. First and foremost one has to trust oneself. That is the hardest thing. We have all been conditioned to one degree or another. We are taught that men act this way and women act that way. We've been taught that this thing or that thing is wrong. If we think about those things, let alone doing them, we feel guilty about it. Being honest with oneself is key to making a relationship last because if you cannot be honest with yourself, you cannot be honest with your partner(s).

For example, I often told myself I was not polyamorous. I denied that I could have interest in anyone outside of my primary relationship. But I did find others attractive and not just in a sexual way. I tried to mitigate those feelings and it proved disastrous to my relationships and it hurt people. It took me years to reconcile myself with that fact, and now my current relationship doesn't have that shadow hanging over it. When you can trust yourself, it is much easier to elicit and maintain the trust of others.

The other thing is that we have a tendency to judge our relationships by common standards. We sometimes forget that we live what is referred to as "an alternative lifestyle." If it is indeed an "alternative" then why do we constantly judge it by mainstream values? This goes back to our conditioning. Our environments, our society, our families and friends have all played a part in the development of our personal norms and standards and sometimes we fail to analyze them and adjust them to the person who we are today and the lives we lead in the here and now. It's as if I grew up in Hawaii but wanted to live the same way in Brooklyn. I'd have to make some adjustments, even if fundamentally I'd be the same person. BDSM requires that we change some of our perspectives and perceptions.

I grew up during the Civil Rights movement with parents who were intent on helping me to understand my history and culture in the midst of the turmoil of the struggles of the times. I learned how to navigate those waters. When I first came upon the BDSM scene, I really didn't feel different, but I know that was because of the first people who I met coming into the scene. It was a good while before I met other Black people into BDSM. Then I became aware of groups that were almost exclusively for People of Color.

In the beginning I was a bit ambivalent. I was glad that there were other people who looked like me and shared my culture and common experience, but at the same time I wondered why they felt the need to segregate themselves from the larger scene. I soon learned the hard way.

There are people who don't see us as people but as a fetish. I get unsolicited requests from "Queen of Spades" looking for BBC* (not the British television network). [ed. - *Big Black Cock] I have been solicited for cuckold fantasies by people who don't know me. I have heard many women of color speak about how they have been approached, some in very menial, vulgar terms, and others who are approached by fetishists thinking they are complimenting them by calling them "Ebony Goddess" and "Nubian Queen." They'll offer service not caring if the woman identifies as submissive, or speak to them in demeaning, racist terms. Even in classes about BDSM there is often little talk if any about the differences between Black skin and white skin in terms of how it reacts. You'll hear presenters talk about "shades of red" and other terms that should be – but seldom are – modified when dealing with darker people.

I know of more than one Black BDSMer who has been mistaken for the only other Black BDSMer the non-black person has heard about. Several Black women with short natural hair have been asked if they are Mama Vi Johnson [ed. - BDSM activist and leatherwoman], in spite of their age, body and complexion differences. I know a Black titleholder who was mistaken for the only Black man known within a particular community. I've seen people make assumptions based entirely upon skin color. Indeed, some of them feel they can tell you not only what to be offended about, but how you should address the offense based on skin color. When a Board member of an organization I belonged to made a remark I felt was racist, another Board member who is also a person of color was asked if it was offensive. When he said no, my point was dismissed.

Time and again, especially in various Internet forums, I have heard Blacks and other People of Color express their sentiments about a racial incident only to be told, "You should use this as an opportunity to teach others," or "Instead of getting upset, why don't you open up a dialogue?" Recent news events have brought out hidden feelings and quite a few Black BDSMers have been shocked by the vitriolic and racist comments made by people we thought were friends, including some alleged pillars of the Community. Plenty of bridges were burned. It's a cold reminder that not everyone considers you a part of their BDSM community. Hopefully we can transcend this but the way the world at large is going today, I know it will take a great deal of time and effort.

Deborah Addington

Scholar, esoteric researcher, ordained minister, writer, and lifestyle dominant, Deborah is renowned for her study of the intersections between BDSM and sacred teachings.

I've always been on the top side. I identify as a dominant and a sadist. I'm not a switch, though I can and have played on both sides. I'll bottom to needles, for example, but for me, it's a pursuit of hedonism and sensation, not a pursuit of the submissive role. I'm not a service top either. I like hurting people. The older I get, the more comfortable I am in my sadism and the more I see myself in service by way of creating intense, body-based spiritual experiences for the people with whom I play. Dominance and submission are inextricably linked; we all have both urges in us. The trick is in choosing how to play out one's tendencies in reality.

I believe BDSM saved my life. If I hadn't discovered healthy, consensual outlets for my natural inclinations, I would have gone through life entirely as a raging shitfuck asshole. You know the type. It's that person who always has something to prove and needs to be dominant in every situation. BDSM provides an appropriate context that renders my impulses and tendencies a gift I can offer to others without causing them – or me – harm.

My BDSM life today is complex. I am married (thirteen years together), and separated. My wife was my slave for 7 years. I have a friend who says that she never breaks up with anyone; they just shift their relationships into more appropriate forms. I'm in the middle of doing that now. I have lovers and playmates, as well as a few service relationships currently. I train people in how to pay attention and I serve as a mentor. The service I receive facilitates my life; training others to serve enhances their lives. It's a lovely win-win.

There's nothing inherently right or wrong about BDSM; people have always done kinky things with/to/for each other. BDSM is about finding a context that permits safe expression of socially rejected proclivities and refusing to be defined by others' notions of right and wrong. There's something wrong with a culture that tells us not to be ourselves because they cannot make room for the different or the novel. As Krishnamurti put it, "It is no measure of health to be well adjusted to a profoundly sick society." Being kinky outside of appropriate contexts makes humans into jerks. But with appropriate context, people become integrated, more evolved, more decent human beings.

I was surprised when I discovered that BDSM could create ecstatic states. I knew what an ecstatic state felt like; I experienced my first one when I was 9, in a religious context. At 17, I learned that BDSM could get me into what Dossie Easton [*BDSM author and family therapist*] calls the "forever place." Transcendent, ecstatic, and altered states are other names for this ineffable experience. In fact, the reason I went back to grad school was to study the connection between BDSM and spirituality.

I've found that BDSM adapts readily to different stages of life. I'm not 20 anymore; I'm 50. While I remain basically the same pervert I've always been, how those inherent tendencies are expressed shifts over time. It will continue to shift; I cannot imagine becoming invested or embedded in a way of life that was rigid and prohibited change. I want my identity and integrity to remain intact yet still have plenty of room to change and evolve. BDSM does that for me. I've been surprised to see how easy it is to shift and adapt my practices while still sitting comfortably on a lounge chair under the umbrella of BDSM.

Yes, I have leather and toys and have attended many play parties and events. Acquiring those things is a way of flagging in a community to indicate that one is a member. Early on, that's important. But while identifying oneself by externalia may represent inclusion, if it stops there, you become trapped by the trappings. If BDSM is only about dressing up in certain fetish attire, or only doing certain things with certain people in certain environments – all the external components of what we do – then one's BDSM life would end once those things went away or changed. I am no less of a BDSMer today than I was 30 years ago, though some of my practices look a lot different today on the outside.

Professionally, I am an ordained minister and have a Masters of Divinity. I'm working on a PhD in theology, specializing in BDSM, sex and spirituality. My current work is examining BDSM as a spiritual praxis through the lens of Marcella Althaus-Reid's book, *Indecent Theology*. All Abrahamic sacred texts – the Bible, the Torah, the Qur'an – are about power and power imbalanced relationships. At some point, we stopped using the sacred texts as manuals for learning how to live with and among each other, and began using them as weapons to reinforce the authority structures of the dominant paradigm and for determining which behaviors are "right" and "wrong." This is a mistake and a misuse of wisdom. Almost every kinkster I know has "church burns" because of the misuse of sacred texts and bad theology. In my counseling practice, I strive to help people reclaim what they've lost that's worth keeping and release old, bad habits that stem from religion's misapplications. BDSM rituals and practices are often a part of this healing.

I see BDSM activities as a form of communion which hinges on intent. Imagine two people, both of whom are eating crackers and drinking grape juice. If one person is merely having a snack and the other is eating and drinking with intent, as a ritual or sacred act, then those two apparently identical activities become quite different from one another. For some, and most certainly for me, BDSM is a sacred space that helps me make sense of myself and my place in this world and allows me to share stories, rituals, practices and experiences within a community of affinity (a congregation, if you will).

The real challenges in successful BDSM relationships is building communication skills and living from an empowered place of proactive choice instead of fear-based reactivity. Saying, "Oh, I can't be tender because doms don't do that," or "This obedient pose is how I was told submissives must act," is the root of a fear-based choice. Proactivity from an empowered place can afford to look at what really *IS* in that moment and then makes choices in line with oneself and one's desires. BDSM fosters this kind of self-empowerment.

I don't care how many pairs of leather pants or corsets or fancy tools and toys a person has; I care that they know who they are and can share that with me in ways we find mutually satisfying and deeply pleasurable. Without personal integrity, the externals mean nothing, and the depth and duration of any relationship is limited.

Justin Tanis

Theologian, ordained minister, transgender activist, author, and artist Justin is renowned for his decades of work on the connections between sex, gender, theology and the arts.

I'm not exactly sure how I'd identify today. I hope that I still have that same eagerness for physical exploration as I did starting out, but today my needs are tied to intimacy and connection. What I have (and what I love) are relationships in which both people care for and serve one another in complementary ways. We're in a Sir/boy relationship, although, frankly, I don't especially resonate with those words. The best way to describe us is to say that we are a team with equal power and unequal authority, with love and mutual care at the very center of what we do. We just got married because that seemed an important way to care for each other in sickness and in health.

I have been called a slave in the past, but we don't use that word in my current relationship – my partner feels strongly that one cannot own a human being and that to claim to do so violates his personal morality. We both feel strongly called as white people to stand against racism in our society and using the word slave would interfere with that *for us*. We respect others who do use the word, especially African-Americans, but I feel that using the word in a sexualized context can be seen as trivializing the evil that slavery was/is.

For a number of years I lived in complete service, including sleeping for several years in bondage every night in a cell. It was a profound joy to devote myself to service. It's not how I live at the moment but I feel lucky to have been able to experience it. It is a rare thing in this society to say that someone else's needs are worth more than my own; it was a liberating and life-giving experience.

The best surprise in my BDSM journey was finding people who truly live the way that I desired to live. When I was younger, I wondered if it was all just a fantasy and if anyone actually was able to build a life this way. I found out it was real. When I began to meet a lot of other leather folks in the 1990s, I found the masculinity of leathermen profoundly alluring. Yes, it was seriously masculine but also queer; it spoke to me in my transition, and showed me the kind of man I (would) want to be. Leathermen offer a different take on what it means to be a man than our society usually validates – queer men who claim authority, masculine men who give up control and power. I remain deeply grateful to them because they've taught me so much.

My biggest disappointment is when people who seem authentic say, "Oh, don't take all this too seriously, it's just an act." I have learned that it is possible to live your dreams and create the life you want; it is a joy when you find co-travelers on this road who want to do it with you. I am saddened by those who aren't willing or feel unable to do what they need to do to fulfill their desires. I am also disappointed when people say they can never use their real names or be honest about their proclivities outside of the BDSM community. All of us CAN use our names and be out. It simply may not be a good decision for all people to do so (especially those with young children). I still wish people would acknowledge that it is, "a decision that is not right for me at this time," instead of saying, "I cannot." That makes it sound like they have no choice or ownership over their choice to be closeted. Plus, it has felt like mostly straight people who won't take the risk, leaving the burden on us queer people.

I am also extremely concerned about sexism in the M/s community. Given how many men go to professional femdoms, it just doesn't follow that such an incredibly high percentage of the visible dominants at public events are men. This screams sexism to me. In my ideal world, there'd be a much broader range of genders who are dominant and we'd be able to see that genuine variety manifested and respected in our public and private spaces.

I think the Maslow Pyramid is a good way to look at BDSM relationships – are you moving towards higher self-actualization? Are your needs being met? Then good. If you are worried about these things, can you change the relationship to better meet them? This way of living should make us happier, better people. But sometimes our desires can be so strong that we settle for people who meet the outward appearance but not our inner needs. If BDSM isn't making your life better, stop doing it or do it differently.

The BDSM community is good on safety, okay on reality, not excellent on pleasure. Too much of our education is big on technique and low on pleasure and reality, in my opinion. The emphasis on safety is important but it can also inhibit a sense of exploration. Of course people shouldn't be hitting the kidneys, but I think maybe they should feel freer to push their bodies in other ways to fully explore their personal potentials. The really amazing, transcendent BDSM experiences aren't all tidy and safe.

My professional life has included years and years of advocacy for trans people and in many ways, the leather community has been my space away from that. I want to be valued for who I am, what I bring to a scene/relationship, and not what my gender is. I am, however, *incredibly* happy that there are trans people who are passionate about being visible and vocal about being trans in the community. I wish I knew the name of the transwoman who I saw at the APEX dungeon about 10 years ago. She had not had any genital modifications and was beautifully feminine and walked around that dungeon naked with the attitude that she truly belonged there. She has been my role model since then. I hope that she is as confident in her body, in her role as a bottom, and in her space as she seemed that night because she totally rocked it. I am not that confident yet but I'm working on it.

Ministering to LGBT and BDSM people who feel a conflict between sexuality and spirituality must start by questioning why they are experiencing this division and offering ideas on healing that rift. We have to question values and learn how to relate them to our sexuality, often in new ways that we weren't taught as children. So many people learned and deeply absorbed the message that sexual shame contributes to a spiritual life. The opposite is true. One of my favorite classes at the Center for Lesbian and Gay Studies in Religion and Ministry is my course on Sexuality in Sacred Art because it reminds my students and me that sexuality and spirituality have been linked throughout most of human history. For example, the *Song of Songs*, which is the story of two people engaged in sexual pleasure, was the most read and copied book of the Bible during the Middle Ages. Sex was a gateway to spiritual insight and experience for millennia and it can be that for us again.

We have been given bodies capable of profound pleasure in the midst of a creation filled with an awesome array of genders and sexualities. Why would we say it is sinful to engage this capacity rather than recognize it may be sinful to deny it? Why are our theologies and moralities related to sexuality so often rooted in "no, no, no!" rather than in the Golden Rule? A sexual theology that is serious about treating others as we want to be treated offers a much clearer road to moral action. It requires genuine consent, mutual pleasure, respect, and joy, whether it's applied to an hour between near-strangers or a lifetime between committed partners.

This is not to say that anything goes. It is totally worth holding out for the person who makes you insanely, deliriously happy. The intimate details vary widely from person to person but we should all be aiming for emotional, spiritual and sexual satisfaction. I've had great tricks but I've had better long-term relationships. For me, sex in a long-term relationship with the same person has been the most satisfying because it is an ongoing dialogue and source of joy between us. (Damn it, my mother *was* right about that.)

BDSMers 45-

*Robin Young

> *A popular active player in the BDSM/leather scene of the 1990s, Robin was a foundational BDSM educator on UseNet.*

I was 21 years old when first interviewed, and I'm 45 now. Today I identify as 100% switch, confirmed bisexual (though leaning heterosexual), doing less gender bending but still some. I was a programmer then, and am a programmer now. I don't feel that BDSM has changed my views of life in general, as it's been part of my personality since before I was a sexual being. To be accurate, I'd say it's the foundation of my views of life in general. I don't know that I had any expectations, but it has been mostly wonderful all along. Though I used the handle Robin Young in 1993, I now prefer Roderick Grey, a name I picked a decade ago, and nothing to do with that 50 Shades business.

Today I am fifteen years into a heterosexual marriage, with children for the last decade. I was quite polyamorous in my twenties, and throughout the 1990s, but when my biological clock went off at age thirty in the year 2000, I decided to become monogamous. This was entirely the right decision, as very young children are even more incredibly consuming of emotional energy than a primary partner! Now that our children are growing up and nearing adolescence, our marriage is opening up and becoming "monogamish" (hat tip to Dan Savage). This is still an early exploration for us and we are moving cautiously, but so far, so very good.

BDSM has been one of the constants in my life. Having children took me mostly out of the Community for quite a few years, but my wife and I have been kinky in private throughout that time, and we are now rejoining the Community with renewed vim.

Our personal boundary with our children is that our sex life is entirely our personal business, so while we intend to educate our children on the critical importance of consent and on the plethora of sexual behaviors in the world that can be safely enjoyed (with proper preparation), we do not plan to share with them specifically what we do together. That's none of their business. They are nearing adolescence, so these conversations will soon begin in earnest. We have a small room in our home that we keep locked, since that's where all the "inappropriate stuff" is kept – as far as they're currently concerned, that mainly means scary books that Dad enjoys. As they get older and wise up, they'll still be kept out of there!

If I could go back in time, I would've been more discreet online. I published a kinky FAQ for years under my real name. Then Google came along and indexed everything, and I had to come out to my parents as kinky, since apparently my given name is unique on the whole Internet! My kids will probably turn up that old stuff any year now, and that will be a teachable moment that was decades in the making – "Kids, DO NOT use your own name on the Internet unless you want the whole world to know!"

My wife was a BDSM novice when we met, so she took quite a chance on marrying me. Over time I found that I carried a lot of sexual urgency with me, mostly nervousness about whether my dizzying array of fantasies would ever come true. My wife is less kinky than I am (as she would concur), and she has not always been comfortable with everything I wanted. It took us quite a few years to sort these things out, particularly during our monogamous phase. Ultimately I realized that achieving every last one of my own desires was considerably less important than focusing on the many areas where our interests and fantasies aligned. Giving up some of my tension around these issues was one of the most mature things I have ever done.

I never expected my wife to be open to polyamory whatsoever, so I would definitely say that's been a big surprise. It actually is working out very well, as the things I want to do with others are not the things she wants to do, so she is significantly more than okay with it all.

It is also surprising to find myself in much better physical shape than ever before in my life – strength and flexibility training is something that I am surprised every masochist doesn't do, as masochism is basically a superpower when it comes to intense workouts! Every masochist knows that not all pain is bad, and that's critical when it comes to the gym. Learning how to keep myself really fit is paying enormous dividends in my sex life with my wife and with my other play partners, and I expect it to extend my active and satisfying sex life by decades (no small thing now that I'm in my mid-forties).

Today, I look at a lot of the conversation about "rape culture" as being largely about men feeling entitled to having sex when they want it, how they want it, with whomever they want to have it. This kind of entitlement, to me, is toxic both to our society and our relationships. Consent is the linchpin to all successful human interactions. Our society has dismally far to go in really grasping this lesson, though I've seen some hopeful signs of change in just the last year.

Once there are no more drunk girls getting assaulted in fraternities, once everyone knows that Christian Grey in *Fifty Shades of Grey* is actually an abuser and not a consensual BDSM practitioner, once children are no longer getting pressured into sexual situations they are unready for, then I will feel that the BDSM community has achieved its destiny of truly educating the world about the meaning of consent.

slave feyrie

At 37, slave feyrie is the youngest person to meet our criteria of 20+ years experience with BDSM relationships. Under this name she is active in Scene events and community.

I had BDSM experiences as a teenager in high school, but I officially came into the "scene" around my 21st birthday. I identified as a slave, but that term was discouraged and unpopular at that time. Looking back, I was really a bottom who enjoyed feeling submissive, and I sought out partners who evoked those feelings in me.

I am careful about my use of terms because I believe words need to have set meanings. I have seen a lot of pain and heartache in our Community when people use the same word to mean different things. Most famously, as a Community, we are incapable of agreeing on definitions of things. So when I speak publicly or teach classes, I make sure to add, "Not everyone agrees on this definition, but when I speak, this is what I mean." That applies here too.

A Master/slave relationship is a long-term committed relationship where the Master assumes total responsibility for the slave, and the slave offers total obedience and surrender, which may or may not involve SM or sex. M/s is an ideal we work toward in a daily practice, in the way that yoga is a daily practice. Some days you can get your leg over your head and stand on one finger. Some days you can barely sit for 5 minutes. This is what 24/7 M/s is like. So with that preamble, I identify as a slave. I am in a 24/7 live-in Master/slave Owner/property relationship. We are also married, which to us means "legal Ownership."

I guess outwardly, when someone hears the word "slave," without understanding what that means to us, they could jump to some really negative conclusions. I am a Feminist. There is a basic, core concept in Feminist Theory, which views any kind of "power over" relationships as negative. Could my choice to be a slave be a response to my inherent oppression as a woman by the Patriarchy? Sure it could. But my response is, who has the right to dictate how I respond to my oppression? Maybe it empowers me to sexualize it?

The end result is that I am a happy, fulfilled and actualized person with an amazing life. Not only is this my sexuality, this is my spiritual path, and walking that path continually leads me to become a better person. Just like the most beautiful flowers can grow from unlikely compost, BDSM and slavery have bloomed me into a beautiful person with a beautiful life and I am so thankful for them.

One of the biggest revelations BDSM has given me has been the concept of radical honesty with self and others. You can't live or play at this level without radical honesty. Another is that martyrdom buys you nothing but resentment. It is within my nature to sacrifice myself, my well-being, my finances, and my happiness for love.

Today, I think the shadow side of that is the belief that sacrificing myself should "buy" the love of the other person. And really, that is non-consensual. In reality, it also made me less valuable as property and filled me with massive feelings of resentment. I had to learn to stop trying to buy love in that way. To live as a slave, I had to explore any manipulative tendencies in myself and grow out of using them. The biggest obstacle to BDSM relationship happiness is the tendency to "play act" to the point of dishonesty, and trying to create relationships in the image of books, movies, or the preaching of people on the Internet. It leads to ugliness and hurt. Radical self-honesty is the only way to break with this.

Sometimes we say, "You must be this tall to ride," and that is so true in BDSM. You must have your shit together. You have to be really stable, both financially and emotionally, so that you aren't secretly motivated by unmet needs. You have to know what you want and need and exactly how much you can give without becoming an unstable needy mess. You have to know how to fill your own emotional tank. If you rely on someone else to do it for you or to save you from yourself, it won't work. It's also a huge and unfair burden to put on someone else. I speak from 23 years of watching a lot of train wrecks caused by these things.

I've had some lows myself. I gave my trust fund to a former Dominant, only to have him abandon me and use it to fund his wedding to another woman. I was in a really bad poly relationship for 3 years where I was treated really unfairly and emotionally cruelly. I thought there was nothing I could do to remove this toxic person from my life because my choice was either deal with it or lose my Master.

Those experiences forced me to change. I stopped giving of myself so easily. I began taking my financial and emotional well-being as seriously as my physical well-being. With those changes, I also changed my orientation from polyamory to monogamy. I don't think poly is inherently bad but it really REALLY does not work for me. The root of poly is the idea that we do not own each other. The root of M/s is the idea that we do.

Marrying my Master has been a dream come true. It's like being Cinderella. It's like living 20 years in a desert on crickets and suddenly being given a palace full of cake. It was also really hard to transfer from a fantasy relationship where I saw him a few hours a week or a few days at a time to picking up his dirty socks and not being able to "go home" when he pisses me off. It is the most intense, hardest, and most epically awesome thing I have ever experienced.

This is real life for us. We stay grounded through our rituals and protocols. We can be in the most mundane place and there are a thousand things going on between us. I am "i," folding his napkin a certain way, giving him 3 ice cubes in his water glass. I kiss his hand when I greet him. There are a billion little things which remind us of who we are to each other, through death, or birth, or taxes or grocery shopping.

How will this work when I have his child later this year? Obviously we will not expose our child to anything age inappropriate. We will keep the things going on between us between us – in the same way vanilla people continue their relationships when they have children. We have a picket fence too – ours just happens to be wrapped in black leather.

❧ Chapter 5 ☙
Real BDSM Relationships

In 1993 when people first read *Different Loving*, they were learning not only that there were names for the things they fantasized about doing sexually, but that other adults were living out those fantasies safely, sanely, and with mutual respect. They also learned that as long as the kink was mutually consensual, done for mutual pleasure, it was on the gamut of acceptable, normal sexuality.

Today, we can demonstrate that BDSM relationships also lead to successful marriages, blissful partnerships, and great personal satisfaction in the long-term. They rise and fall like non-kinky relationships, and are subject to unexpected changes (whether from a disability, an undiagnosed mental health issue or aging). There are some failures, there are disappointments, there is a learning curve. In the end, though, the durability and positive attitudes that result from long-time BDSM activity have hugely enhanced and fulfilled almost everyone who actively pursued mutually consensual BDSM throughout adulthood.

From the body of interviewees with people who have now been involved in BDSM for 20 years or more, and despite the dissimilarity in some points of view particularly around the organized (clubs, groups, events) side of the scene, four powerful themes resonate throughout:

1. Consensuality is non-negotiable. Mutual respect is a keystone of acceptable BDSM sex.

2. Clear communication and honesty make BDSM relationships flourish.

3. Personal and relationship evolution is part of the lifecycle of BDSM relationships.

4. BDSM relationships engender self-actualization and empower people to embrace their authentic needs.

In this chapter, we draw from the Community pool, to explore an even wider range of information and education about the relationship issues that arise in BDSM.

Successful BDSM relationships

I turned to the Community to find out what they believe makes their own BDSM relationships strong and to see how this larger pool, some of whom are far younger and less experienced than our core group of interviewees, compared. On the whole, the same themes emerged – mutual consent and mutual respect; commitment to communicating about the sex, the relationship and the agreed roles; the maturity and flexibility to accept change; and the rewards of living one's own truth in bonded relationships. A few people also added the importance of strong sexy physical chemistry.

What do you see as the keys to a successful BDSM relationship?

RB: I value the trust we have with each other and the tight bond that comes from all the shared experiences, rituals, and the fact that both of us actively make our relationship a priority. To keep an active power exchange going for years takes both of us committed to working on the relationship regularly and this means that our relationship works a lot like a hobby we share. Other couples may tinker with cars together. We tinker with our relationship. It rarely gets a chance to be ignored, taken for granted, or treated as a lower priority.

TJE: The mutual acceptance that this relationship is work, work we both must be willing to do. The decision that our relationship will be a safe-space for each of us to be ourselves. None of that could have happened if we hadn't known ourselves fairly well before coming together. We had to have separate journeys before we could walk this road together. In our case we also have been blessed by another family member who, while he does not have a Ds dynamic with us, is very supportive of us as we are. In short, what makes a good BDSM relationship, is what makes a good relationship.

FM: Working equally hard at it, communication, transparency, having lots of other hobbies, really liking each other, trust, confidence, (not being needy), empowerment, compersion (poly), listening, sharing, trying new things, frequent laughter, not taking your 'role' too seriously, being generous and giving as much as you get.

AL: SSC [Safe, Sane, Consensual]. No jealousy! Open and safe communication. Safe word respect. A desire to fulfill each other's needs with an understanding of compromising on limits. Love. Friendship. Adventure. Spontaneity. Role play. Trust to keep each other safe from/with others, and the knowledge we've got each other's back for our deepest dark secrets, no matter what. (An understood gag order if you will.) *Never fight dirty!* After 29 years of marriage, the importance of revisiting our 'contract' and fine tuning it to reflect changing needs, wants, desires, goals, and fantasies. Understanding if the other can't fulfill a *need* we have their permission to fulfill it elsewhere.

ACL: Allowing myself to be completely open and vulnerable in communication with my partners is where I start. We establish boundaries and communicate when those boundaries need to be adjusted back or expanded. We have complete respect for each person as an individual and do not go into a scene with a one size fits all expectation. Trust is a must and if there is ever any wavering, communication again is key. Long-term partners are irreplaceable, yet we find it healthy to mix things up at times by including others with similar interests.

NED: Open communication, trust, respect, a good sense of fun, love, friendship, acceptance.

KB: COMMUNICATION, trust, honesty and oh yeah – COMMUNICATION!

AL2: The depth of the relationship, finding out *why* we might enjoy X, what underlies it. Why my partner likes being beaten is more important to me than simply taking it at face value. I guess that is communication, but it is in-depth communication. Asking and learning the hard questions of each other.

MW: My owner's willingness to work out our issues and difficulties, my willingness to forgive both of us, and our continued wonderment and gratitude for one another. I sought him for over two decades, he sought me for twice as long. Despite our differences, we are so much stronger as a unit that we embrace even the trials and travails. It is truly something to be able to live a life you assumed would be relegated to the realm of fantasy because your hopes outstripped any possible reality. We are both fortunate, and we live that every day.

ACL: Freedom, vulnerability, and equality which seems ironic given the nature, but for us, despite a very "I am the boss" relationship, both of us feel equal to the other, more so than any other relationship. (That could just be us rather and not the dynamic, I don't know.)

MF: Pure sexual chemistry and strong mutual physical attraction are some specific qualities that help us make our kink so good.

JD: POWER, obedience, respect, affection, fun, creativity, adrenaline.

AH: Trust, learned rituals, and dedication.

AL: Pleasure! I have a huge mind fuck guilt complex issue from my conservative upbringing. He gets it and respects it. So his secret wicked smile is enough to charge me up.

WH: I believe that the same things that make any relationship a good one have to be there in a lifestyle one for it to be a good one.

It goes without saying, but it's good people said it anyway, that mutual attraction is as important in BDSM as in any other type of relationship. That attraction, however, is often larger than the physical characteristics or accouterments that typically draw people together. For BDSMers, attitude, open-mindedness, commitment, honesty and positive energy may be as seductive, if not more so, than physical beauty.

BDSM and romantic love

Because of old mental health myths, abiding cultural inhibitions about non-conformist sex, and all the mass-market novels about BDSM (whether *Story of O* or anything else) which make love and consent seem irrelevant in BDSM, the place of romantic love in BDSM has been massively misunderstood and misconstrued. The dark Sadean shadow – that sadomasochists are victims and abusers – hangs over us still. The public commonly assumes that people who enjoy weird or kinky sexual pleasures have personal problems and emotional complexes that prevent them from knowing true love.

One of the most common misconceptions I hear as a therapist, is the partner of a fetishist who feels threatened by the fetish, and believes that "(s)he loves the outfit/gear more than (s)he loves me." They ask, "Why aren't I enough, why does there always have to be a toy or outfit?" It is undeniably difficult for a non-kinky person to feel the same way about BDSM/fetish as someone who may well have BDSM/fetish in their DNA. And it must be noted that mentally unstable people who are also fetishists create tsunamis of pain in their relationships by dint of their instability. But grounded, mentally healthy BDSMers don't actually want their fetish more than they want a happy relationship, they want their fetish in the context of a happy relationship.

The cliché that BDSMers are more interested in their toys than their partners is also partly an outgrowth of the BDSM social environment, which accommodates newcomers and sexual adventurers, along with all the partners of people who rejected them for their kinks (see above), and who seek outlets for their needs in the BDSM community. The BDSM community has long been a general repository for people who feel sexually isolated and alone with their kinks. So experimentation with toys, mentoring, demonstrations of techniques and equipment, and all manner of non-sexual acts and role playing are common sights in public spaces, as are people parading their interests without inhibition. Hedonists and thrill seekers swell the BDSM ranks for activities such as bondage/rope suspensions and Shibari [ornate Japanese-inspired bondage], just as pagans and seekers have flooded into the body modification side of BDSM, seeking paths to ecstasy through sadomasochistic body rituals. To an outsider looking in, the open embrace of kinky activity may look like sexual permissiveness on the surface. It is permissive in the sense that "your kink is (usually) okay." It is not, however, an orgy or sexual free-for-all. There is very low tolerance for non-consenting behaviors, including touching people without their permission or trying to join in an activity without an invitation or explicit consent.

The scene has always accommodated the needs of solitary players. At first, it was because there was an atmosphere of fear and shame that kept most people in the closet. A trip to a club might be their only opportunity to have any kind of BDSM conversation or action in their lives. Depending on where and how you live, this may still apply – play parties and dungeon events remain a vital outlet for people who, for whatever reason, have not found a compatible BDSM partner. Professional dominants looking for new clients, activists and educators who love teaching/mentoring, and poly/swing or other libidinous strangers are usually available to lend a hand (or whip) to lonely newbies. Safe words, safe signals, dungeon monitors, and other common safety protocols in BDSM settings were intentionally designed to help strangers or near-strangers explore BDSM without causing harm.

So what about love? Do BDSMers experience romantic love like other people do? Or does purely pleasure seeking behavior dominate their relationships?

I asked the Community if love was important to their relationships.

What do think about the role of love in BDSM relationships?

NED: I'm so glad for this question. So many vanillas think that we kinky people are emotionally/mentally fucked up and are incapable of loving others. That simply isn't true. Love is the basis of my relationship with my Master.

SM: I think you sometimes see this in people who are into kink but with less experience, perhaps before they experience a deep loving kink relationship first hand. I love my sub very deeply, in a for-the-rest-of-my-life kind of way. We've had some discussions about the preconceived ideas he had about love in a relationship because his previous experience was limited to physical-only partners.

RB2: I find that many vanillas seem to have the misconception that all BDSM relationships are superficial, temporary, and two-dimensional, only focused on sex and play. The fantasy is that we're all constantly getting laid with a buffet of casual freaky partners and little emotional attachment. The challenge is showing that this isn't always the case without losing any of our sex positive message or slut shaming those who do enjoy plenty of casual fun with an array of consenting partners.

AL: Vanilla. Huh. You mean the true-love-waits-sex-for-procreation lie vanilla population? Seriously. There are a lot of loving kink couples! Some proudly married 20-40 years. We've been married since 1986. But we are a silent populace because of laws and closed minded people. We don't want to lose our kids, jobs, or social standing. I live in Florida, where it is illegal for an unmarried male and female to live at the same residence! Once, at a Linux (computer code language) conference my husband and I got called out for my Kindle and Google library and history. My husband looked at me because I had dressed for him, and said, "I knew I forgot something. I should have remembered your collar and leash, Kitten." Don't think I've seen so many fish mouths at once. Then again I got tons of email thanking me for our bravery.

ACL: I want government and religion to get out of our business. Individuals need to be allowed to form partnerships and marriages that fulfill them. I have found people in the BDSM and poly community to be well-adjusted, intelligent and socially responsible.

ZBL: I think some of the confusion comes from conflating BDSM with swinging. Many muggles seem to think that what we do is all based around sex.

MM: Some kinky folks want partners. Some kinky folks want props. Some kinky folks want both. One of the things I think is critical to examine in any pair-bonded relationship: what is more important to you, the relationship itself or the forms the relationship takes? If your D/s relationship falters, are you more concerned about losing the pair bond or the power exchange?

RS: There are certain relational requirements to succeed in the BDSM social scene. It helps to take personal responsibility, to be able to negotiate, to desire, or at least tolerate, seeing others naked and sexual and being seen naked and sexual yourself. Straight people fear stigmatization, and imagine that our strategies to avoid it – using avatars and scene names, or leading double lives – must interfere with or diminish our intimacy. They assume there will be intimacy in heteronormative relationships because they expect to find it there, but they don't understand the intimacy that BDSM can provide. With BDSM, you can never know the potential for intimacy unless you jump down the rabbit hole.

ACL: For me, BDSM, power, poly, and swinging do not need to be separated into neat little pockets. I prefer to mix everything up and make uninhibited art. I love to unzip my partner and service their soul. Everyone's secret self is so unique and I like to open each other up so everyone gets the release they desire. I am submissive by nature, but I am just as thrilled to switch things up.

Race Bannon: For me, and I believe many others, some form of love is essentially a prerequisite for really good BDSM.

I also asked the Community to share some of their favorite first encounters with BDSMers.

Do you have any fond memories or stories about BDSM meetings you'd like to share?

PR: I cranked up my courage, strapped on my nine inch heels, and headed out to a nearby play party, hopeful but realistic. Barely in the door, I was saying hello to some friends when I stepped backwards onto someone's play bag and fell... right into the arms of the most handsome butch woman! As I stammered my apologies, she smiled at me, still in her arms, and cooed that it had been her plan all along. Not only did we play that night, but continued to do so for the next six months! I still think of her fondly!!

KPL: First time at a dungeon, the Powerexchange in San Francisco, many moons ago. I was 19, just discovered the Internet and suddenly realized that what I was feeling had a name. That name was Tony. I don't know if she was a transgender or transvestite but the gender she was identifying was female. It was my first time meeting someone like her as well. She was fascinating to me, and I lingered around her stall. She was kindness and generosity personified. She was patient and started a conversation with me, let me hang out with her most of the night and even played with me a little bit. She took my ignorance in stride and helped me learn a few things, instead of chiding or being angry. She kind of set the bar for how newbies should be treated for me. Her kindness is still being paid forward.

CMM: In 2003, I was on the Volunteer Staff for a winner of the Dyke Diva/Dyke Daddy Contest in San Francisco. I was on a journey from years of evolving from bottom to masochist to submissive to slave to submissive to bottom, coming back out nearly the same way I had begun many years prior. After the contest, I accompanied the new title holder Diva to the play party at The Scenery. We had a great time! After bottoming fun, I excused myself in search of protein. I was mid-level flying.

As I exited the main dungeon floor into the hallway, I heard the sweetest melodic voice say, "The Lord is my shepherd; I shall not want. He maketh me to lie down in green pastures: he leadeth me beside the still waters..." I stopped dead in my tracks, sure I had heard the voice of an angel.

I slowly turned back at the doorway and saw her, a sprite of a breathtaking femme, sitting on a stool talking with someone. Our eyes met and exploded. She smiled and cooed slowly, "Well, hey there, Daddy," her grin dancing into my heart and life forever. My heart leapt within me: "I'm a Daddy!!!!" And so, a Leather Daddy was born.

We stayed up all night talking, and she was mine for nearly 3 years and changed who I am forever. To be so adored, to be so loved, so utterly and completely, just as I am... I will always be grateful. I will never forget her, my submissive, my wild and beautiful angel; and I know she is still with me, always. (She passed just two years after we ended our relationship.)

ER: This goes back a couple of decades now. I had known this dominant woman online in BDSM chat for a while. I even met her for drinks once with her fiancé when I was traveling on business in her hometown. And then, lo and behold, I found out she moved to my hometown and had written a BDSM book. When I heard she would be signing copies at a bookstore, I went and asked for her autograph. She remembered me and we talked until somehow I developed the courage to ask her out to a fancy steakhouse for dinner. She said yes. It turned out to be an incredible dinner; we hit it off so well, and talked so deeply, we didn't notice the place was closing around us until the waiters starting hovering. And so began a wonderful F/m relationship. It was the most fulfilling relationship of my life and our friendship has survived more than two decades. I have always considered myself the luckiest submissive male in the world to have served her. She remains my best friend forever.

GW: Let's see... on my first day at my new job in a conservative town, I noticed this one teal-colored car with a rainbow bumper sticker in the parking lot that was there every day. I mustered up my courage and left a note under the windshield wiper on National Coming Out Day, and soon there was a note back under my windshield wiper, and soon my officemates were wondering where I disappeared to every lunch hour as my newfound friend and I struck up an outrageous flirtation.

She couldn't date me right away though as her triad was polyfidelitous. But one day she called and said, "I have good news and bad news! The bad news is that I'm moving out of state. The good news is that my triad is now open to dating others." Breathlessly I replied, "How soon can you come over?" and we began a lovely BDSM dating relationship that continues to this day, albeit long distance. She is now a he, by the way.

Then there's the story of my first BDSM scene ever. I'd been childhood best friends with this person, and we then went our separate ways in our teens. But one day I was back home from college and we ran into each other on a hot New York City August night. We went for Carvel's lemon and lime ice cream and returned to my parents' empty house and caught up on our lives. She was missing her boyfriend who was away for the summer, and she began stretching and sighing and saying how horny she was. Then: "Do you ever have dreams... you know... about women?"

Well, I'd come out as bisexual at college that year, and told her so, and after she got over her indignation that I hadn't come out to her sooner, she continued, "Do you remember how we used to play house as kids?" Oh yes I did – complete with spankings. We lost no time getting upstairs to the bedroom, and spent several happy hours spanking and caressing each other to orgasm. Alas, it was a short lived reconnection – I ran away from home the following week, and her boyfriend returned from his summer away and married her, and the next time I saw her she was quite the proper monogamous lady and no longer into the games of yore.

ST: I went to a house play party and was watching a first time couple walk around and looking a bit lost. Everyone was quite nice to them, but mainly absorbed in doing their own things. I decided to talk to the couple and find out more. They let me know that they had only played at home and were now looking for like-minded individuals. I asked the husband what it was that they liked to do. I saw the confusion on their faces. They asked if I would help and show them some stuff. So I placed her in a blindfold and proceeded to work her up with clothes pins and sensory stimulation.

At one point I stepped off and let her husband take over. He continued to play with her, eventually giving her some very intense pleasure. I was leaning over her husband's shoulder telling her what I was going to do next, while her husband actually did it. The whole time, she thought it was me. When she finally calmed down, still in her blindfold, she exclaimed loudly, "You need to teach my husband how to do that!" I pulled off the blindfold and told her I already did.

She broke down into tears kissing, sobbing and hugging her husband. They both seemed to forget everyone else was in the room. I returned a little later and they were both still there curled up cuddling. It makes me smile to this day thinking about that.

Stay safe and set boundaries

You may have heard that BDSM is dangerous. It is, but not the way the public at large tends to see it. BDSM is dangerous in the hands of dangerous people. True, certain activities carry risk, but the whole point of BDSM education is to demonstrate that those risks can be mitigated by safety protocols and specialized safety techniques (for example, quick ways to release people from bondage in case of emergency). Every professionally manufactured BDSM toy can bring pleasure without harm when used properly. Indeed, for a majority of players, the toys and gear are primarily props to stimulate and delight each other.

Sane people start slowly. It may seem sexier to leap spontaneously into BDSM with a willing partner. Unfortunately, spontaneity without safety protocols or clear-set limits is the culprit behind most BDSM accidents and injuries. As our interview with Fakir Musafar, now 85, showed, you can spend 70+ years enjoying extreme sensations without harm.

You may compare the BDSM learning curve to tightrope walking. You don't start on the high-wire. You begin by practicing low to the ground until you have perfected your balance and developed the skills necessary to move to the next level, and you always use a safety net. The same is true whether you're in a dominant role or a submissive role. A person who picks up a whip or paddle for the first time and proceeds to use it full-force is not only a fraud, but a dangerous, possibly sociopathic fraud. Conversely, a submissive who surrenders power to anyone without first establishing trust and safety is asking for trouble.

Apart from risky behaviors with the gear, though, there are complicated interpersonal issues that can lead to problems and emotional damage. BDSM sexuality does not exempt anyone from the full range of normal human emotions, good, bad and in-between. While classic and popular BDSM fiction – in literature and online – depicts improbably sex-obsessed caricatures who live their roles 24/7 without any wrinkles, in real life, BDSM women get cranky when they get their periods and BDSM men get flustered when they don't get the erections they expected to get, just like everyone else.

BDSMers strive to integrate the knowledge that we're all flawed human beings with human personal relationships. Understanding that your partner is not a one-dimensional character out of the script in your head but a complex and layered human being is critical to the process. Accommodating changes as a natural part of life and BDSM is too. So is accepting that a power relationship doesn't exist between people until they both: (a) want it, (b) negotiate it, and (c) mutually consent to its terms.

BDSM goes wrong when people don't negotiate consent, when they don't discuss their personal likes and dislikes, and when they commit to power relationships without fully understanding what they're getting into. People can be deeply hurt when they buy into the fantasies that pornography and the Internet have stoked. People who are not self-aware enough to set good boundaries with other people; people who do not recognize the difference between consensual BDSM and abuse, aggression or manipulation; and people who pigeonhole others instead of getting to know them as complex individuals, are all generally unfit for functional BDSM relationships – or any other.

This is the real rub: the emotional pain of a dysfunctional BDSM relationship can be as significant and scarring as a physical injury. The bond between people who have made themselves naked and vulnerable to one another is intensely emotional. Whether real or imagined, that bond can do as much harm to vulnerable, unprepared individuals as it can bring joy and satisfaction to those who have done the work. As several of our interviewees pointed out, people who get trapped by roles and hung up on labels miss the whole point of BDSM and, in so doing, often end up bitterly disappointed by their relationships.

Yet tens of millions of people around the world live out their BDSM fantasies in happy, romantic relationships. How have they avoided and overcome all the pitfalls to solid BDSM relationships?

I asked the Community to share their thoughts on red flags that suggest someone is a bad candidate for a good BDSM relationship.

What would be a total deal-breaker for you in a BDSM re-lationship? Is there any one (or three) things you cannot and will not accept?

TA: Actually, I can't think of any way it would be any different than any other close relationship, be it friendship or romantic. Things like stupidity, lack of discretion, poor hygiene, Republican politics, etc. I joke, but EVERY relationship has its roots in TRUST.

KK: Lying and trust were the two biggest ones that came to mind. If you can't trust your play partner(s) will not unreasonably cross your boundaries, it is difficult to continue to take your play to higher levels. Similarly, with lying (especially in the pathological varieties), you lose respect, confidence and often faith in that individual. Liars can also cloak ill intent (and sometimes psychopathic tendencies) such as is seen with the "creepy Dom/Dommes" who take advantage of their sub(s) and then say things like they didn't realize that what was happening wasn't part of the scene.

WA: Lies.

GA: Permanent damage.

RM: Lies/dishonesty.

JW: Lies and Republicans.

RM: Dishonesty and jealousy.

SW: Lying in any form.

RZ: Dishonesty.

MBB: Definitely dishonesty; it's been that experience that has made it difficult for me to enter another relationship for several years now.

KC: Someone who wouldn't respect boundaries. I can be very kinky but there are a few things I am not into – nipple clamps, blood play, extreme edge play and anything involving needles/sharps. Not my thing. Jealousy is another huge no.

JG: Refusal to establish a safeword. 'Asparagus!' is an especially nice one. :) Or refusing to acknowledge a safeword when used.

MM: Own your shit! Everything else can be worked through, worked out, or worked around, but if you can't own your shit there's nothing I can do. ("Own your shit" means, basically, that you know what you're doing and you're willing to admit to whatever it is. You don't have to apologize. Own your shit applies to the good and the bad. You just have to be able and willing to do clear self-analysis.)

HE: Dishonesty, abuse, refusing to talk things through.

ESC: Lying, cheating, and not respecting boundaries.

CM: Dishonesty in all forms (including withholding), violation of boundaries and/or consent (including with others), narcissism and/or extreme selfishness, silent treatment/gaslighting/or any other form of emotional and/or mental abuse, refusal to communicate, lack of empathy for others. Oh, could I go on!

ST: The following come readily to mind: triangulation that includes an individual whose partner is unaware they are engaged in a BDSM relationship with someone else, slipshod hygiene practices, claiming to be emotionally ready to submit but trying to script what their dominant will do, or use/abuse of any illicit drug or alcohol during a session.

LM: Drug addiction, active alcoholism, racism, sexism, cheating on a spouse, physical abuse against spouse or children.

DA: Persistent boundary violations, especially those resulting in emotional, verbal or physical abuse. Abrogation of integrity. Lack of transparency.

ZLC: Do NOT fucking out me. Do not fuck with those closest to me, in other words, do not cause them undue stress. Do not try to manipulate me.

RGH: Non-consent is my number one deal breaker. No means NO.

FM: A person unable and unwilling to be honest and transparent is number one. A person who is so insecure that I have to constantly give them reassurance. A person unwilling to give as much to the relationship as I do.

SS: There are many things that would be a deal breaker for me in any relationship, but these are the ones specific to a BDSM relationship with a primary: 1. Over emphasis on service submission (I don't do windows), 2. No vaginal intercourse, and 3. Abuse of any kind.

DB: 1. Inability to respect boundaries and consent, 2. Refusal of self-care... physical, emotional, psychological. (We all have issues but don't use me, or my play, to "work shit out." I'm not a therapist, nor is BDSM therapy.), and 3. Drug use/drinking while playing.

CM2: What stands out for me right now: 1. Living up to their own values and what they need to be healthy, 2. Respect / Accepting my values (social justice, love of family, maintaining pre-existing and vanilla friendships, etc.). I'm open to discussing anything and reassessing priorities, but just because I'm submissive doesn't mean that I'll let anyone change me in these ways, and 3. Humor and fun. We don't have to be always joking and laughing, but without a sense of humor, we probably wouldn't survive the tough times. Actually, we probably wouldn't get together in the first place.

It's safe to conclude from the above that trust issues are the single greatest obstacle to a good BDSM relationship. While trust, mutual respect, commitment and transparency are important in all intimate relationships, when you add the intense physical experiences and the intense emotional engagements of BDSM, most people will agree that we hold to a higher standard because we have to.

Ethical BDSM

As we pointed out at the beginning of the book, one of the great ironies in late 20th and early 21st century sex research and science is that the more BDSM/fetish behaviors are studied, the more we have data which contradicts the old thinking about why people enjoy this kind of sex and how their sexual identity plays out in real life. From the first time sadomasochism was separated from other types of sex and organized under the label of pathology in the psychiatric literature in the 1880s, and for more than a century after, it was assumed that something was psychologically and morally wrong about people who had orgasms in unconventional, non-heteronormative (i.e., not missionary position) sex.

We now have numerous studies supporting the idea that BDSM enhances a person's psychological and emotional well-being. Consensual BDSM – and particularly the communication required to safely channel BDSM/fetish desires – also reduces the likelihood of interpersonal abuse. There are now psychological and sociological studies which have concluded that BDSMers are as mentally healthy as anyone else, and perhaps more so; and there are medical studies suggesting that sexual behaviors and preferences, gender identity, and the inclinations towards sadomasochistic sex are all encoded in our DNA. We also have a community of scholars and researchers, CARAS (Community-Academic Consortium for Research on Alternative Sexualities, https://carasresearch.org/) devoted to promoting research into alternative sexualities and disseminating results to mental health professionals, the public, and BDSM/fetish communities.

I was curious to know what BDSMers think about their own ethics and morality, and whether they believe BDSM has positively impacted their take on morality. Did their realities agree with the data that BDSM produces happier, more ethical people?

I asked the Community:

Do you think BDSM has impacted your personal morality? Or is morality itself an outdated concept?

SC: In my humble opinion, without morals (and I fully realize that they differ from person to person), our society is fucked... And to answer your question: I am "more moral" since becoming more involved. And a much better communicator.

RB: I think it depends on what you consider morality. I have shed a lot of the "morality" I was raised with, which was based on religious upbringing. In its place, I have embraced ideas surrounding consent, both in my sex life and in everyday life. I've also become more open and accepting of differences, seeing that as a virtue. My morals are based more now on empathy than they are on rules handed down in a book. I try to treat people with compassion, regardless of how they are different from me.

RJ: I've become more conscious of my moral values and maybe refined some of my thinking. I also think we need to take back the word "morality" from the right-wing Christianists who want to monopolize it and call everyone who disagrees with them immoral. We see every day how immoral their behavior is – we should call them on it. I am a moral person. An atheistic, kinky, queer, anarchist moral person.

FS: I think I am more moral than I would have been because of BDSM. BDSM led me to the leather community where being direct and honest, not bullshitting, is a desired trait. I was raised to beat around the bush and expected to manipulate rather than identify and state my needs. BDSM has made me less full of shit. It has made me more transparent. It has made me aware of the primacy of consent. It has made me a champion and fighter when something is unjust rather than a scared sheep. It has made me more accepting of myself and others. I don't think that it makes EVERYONE more moral, or that it is a requirement for morality, but it certainly has made me a better person.

AL2: I think I'm more moral now than I was in my early 20's. I don't know if that's due to BDSM or just getting older and wiser. I'm much less judgemental and more respectful of people around me regardless of their preferences. I like what FS said, "BDSM has made me less full of shit." I feel that applies to me also.

WH: When I was actively involved in a munch and other groups, I think that I took advantage of the opportunities for sex just for sex's sake. That made me feel less moral. Now that I'm not as involved in the groups and sex is not as big a part of it, I believe that it has little effect on my morality.

FG: Less biased. More self-aware. Not necessarily more moral.

VL: Yes. More – or at least more able to express my morality. No, it isn't outdated. The term has been co-opted and corrupted but the concept is still valid.

LM: Yes to some of what has been said. I am a different kind of moral now. It involves no compromise and gentle, steadfast truth-telling.

AL: It enabled me to throw away conservative ingrained socially acceptable morals, and become more moralistic. To become faithful not religious. Different strokes for different folks as long as it's safe, sane and consensual! However you define that.

SM: I think BDSM broadened my vocabulary and gave me permission to communicate my moral convictions on things.

JBL: I think it's expanded my concept of morality from simple child-like black and white extremes to a more complex and nuanced understanding. It's certainly made me more thoughtful of morality in my interactions, which is certainly a positive thing.

RS: The concept of morals will never be outdated. BDSM has made some of the nuances of my morality more complex and situational.

MC: Hard to say how much of that is BDSM itself and how much of it is you and how you would develop in any field. But I do agree that making some of these deeply primal urges conscious – slowing them down and experiencing them with another live person, and doing it safely – gives a person the chance to act more thoughtfully and hence morally in everyday life.

EW: As a kinkster I am *so much more* moral. You cannot dissemble if you're going to have fun and stay safe.

DDK: Whipping men has made me more intuitive, more compassionate, and more able to trust others.

PT: I've become a more moral and ethical person in my 20+ years in the scene.

MW: I think my involvement forced me to stand more steady in my higher self than I had to when I was younger.

GG: A big increase for me as I learn more about sex positive culture.

TJE: One of the things that drew me to BDSM – as in recognizing my place in the Community – was the morality and ethics. The Community's ideals matched my own fairly well.

RJ: I have a much more sophisticated understanding of the Golden Rule than before. "What you would have them do unto you," is a lot more complicated than it sounds.

DM: It has most definitely enhanced and fine-tuned my already fairly well interpreted morals.

AL3: I absolutely feel that my involvement in BDSM and the kink/poly communities has made me a more morally conscious person. In learning and pushing each other's boundaries, in pushing ourselves further together, you must respect the totality of your partner and give them a safe space. Once you learn to respect that what you do has an effect on other people, you learn to think about how you affect ALL other people, and begin to make conscious choices regarding it. We learn to communicate. We learn to be transparent. We learn to accept fully and love fully. Every partner I have, everyone I play with, every client who walks into my dungeon is treated as a whole person, I must accept them as they are and give them a safe space to express – and I find that the more and more people I meet, the more I find myself in love with the beauty and diversity of the world, and accepting and respecting it for what it is.

DRB: I've learned the truth about morality and have grown in leaps and bounds!

FM: In your life you have to choose how important moral introspection and authenticity are for you as a person. BDSM may be catalytic for some people but I don't believe it is inherently so. In my experience you have the same mixture in kink as in non-kink in terms of morality, behaviors, mental illness, etc. I'm relatively introspective with a lifelong interest in behavior mechanics. I care about the quality of life, including sexuality. However, when morality is 'judging' it moves into opportunities to justify violence against others (an immoral state) so it is fair to say I observe my morality very carefully.

KKD: I think I am more moral. I've learned to communicate much better and ask for what I want and need better (and the difference between the two), which in turn has led to being more honest and clear about my actions. This is probably a direct correlation to my involvement in the Community (classes, etc.), but is also a product of maturity (18 years since I discovered this world).

JR: I feel more moral but not morally superior. The "journey to the authentic self" has helped to clarify many positions for me. As my mother used to say, "The truth is easier to remember."

KD: I consider morality to be imposed by society and ethics to be my own self-imposed code of conduct. This has been a long strange journey and I have learned a lot about myself. I would have to say that I am probably more ethical, but less moral (by my definitions). I am also more open and accepting of diversity. I do abhor the word 'tolerance' in the context of differences. I might tolerate a blister if I get one on my foot, but I don't embrace and accept it. Personally, I would rather be embraced and accepted over simply being tolerated any day.

HSM: BDSM requires the utmost honesty and candor. If you enter into the world with a hidden agenda nothing but trouble is in store for you.

JM: I don't think my morality has changed all that much... but my ethics have definitely been improved.

In summary, ethics matter, establishing moral boundaries matter, and it's up to the individual whether they can utilize the lessons learned from safe, sane, consensual BDSM to forge better lives.

ℬ The Proof Is In the Living ℭ

As of this writing, it has been 24 years since we first set out to write a book that explained BDSM as a normal human phenomenon. The authors of this volume will be celebrating their 27th wedding anniversary in 2016, and can report that, like the hundreds of people we interviewed and queried in this book, our lives also reflect the body of testimony by those who believe their lives are more authentic, their sexual happiness is greater, their relationships more profoundly bonded, and their sense of overall well-being vastly enhanced by living true to their sexual needs and desires. If we could go back to the editor who once scorned our assertion that BDSM and love go hand in hand, we could now show her scientific proof.

As shame and contempt for sexual variations have receded in culture, as sex science shows that sexual diversity is a true normal for adults, BDSMers have been increasingly free to define happiness for themselves. The aggregate of the interviews we conducted, all the studies we reviewed, and the hundreds of people we spoke with while researching this new volume, provide a powerful testament to the healthy love and passion possible among BDSMers.

BDSM has EVERYTHING to do with love. Being sexually different isn't wrong. Being sexually different isn't "worse" than being sexually conventional. Being sexually different opens the door to authenticity and to a life lived on one's own terms.

Dr. Gloria G. Brame and William D. Brame
2015

ꙮ Appendix ꙮ
Who's Who in
Different Loving Too

The original different lovers

The authors first began work on *Different Loving* in 1990. All three authors (Brame, Brame, and Jacobs) conducted the interviews in person, by phone, or by correspondence between 1991 and 1992.

Many of our interviewees are out of the closet BDSMers who educate or participate in BDSM culture, their names known widely within the Community. Those designated as "private players" maintain a shield of privacy around their BDSM identities to protect their family relationships and professional lives.

From 2014-2015, Brame and Brame collected 19 interviews from the original participants, and added 12 new in-depth interviews to round out the mix. The 31 individuals are listed below.

19 original interviewees

Alexis deVille: Long-time private player, dominatrix, and transwoman..

Carter Stevens: Founding father of the 1970s porn cinema revolution, prolific porn director and BDSM publisher, and adult movie star (as Steven Mitchell), Carter was inducted into the AVN Hall of Fame in 2009.

Cléo Dubois: BDSM mentor, educator, founder, "Cléo Dubois Academy of SM Arts" and one of the most respected voices in the SM community on the intersections between dominance and spiritual energy. Married to Fakir Musafar.

Constance-Marie Slater: Former owner and founder of "Dressing for Pleasure (US)" boutique and fetish fashion pioneer in the United States. Owner and organizer of the annual International Dressing for Pleasure fetish balls in New York (1980s - 1990s).

Dian Hanson: Fetish magazine and book editrix extraordinaire, promoting sex-positive information and social acceptance of fetishism, now the power behind Taschen Books.

Eve Howard: Co-founder and co-owner of Shadow Lane, one of the oldest and most successful spanking fetish companies. The Shadow Lane social media network has been one of the primary organs of the spanking scene for the past twenty-five years. There are currently twelve titles in the Shadow Lane novel series and the reboot of the company's flagship magazine *Stand Corrected*, went to press in the summer of 2015.

Fakir Musafar: Performance artist, teacher, and one of the founders of the modern primitive and body modification movements. Founder and Director of Fakir Intensives. One of the world's most respected presenters and educators on the intersection of body ritual and modification and spirituality. Married to Cléo Dubois.

Gerrie Blum: Aka Lady Gillian, long-time scene player, bisexual activist and, with her husband Mitch Kessler, former publisher and long-time BDSM toy seller.

Baby Glenn: A private BDSM player, Glenn's diaper fetish helped him cope with disability.

James: Aka James W in the original volume, withdrew from BDSM when his Mistress/slave relationship ended.

Kiri Kelly: Private player, former fetish model and star of sweetly sensational spanking films for adults.

Lady Elaina: Known as Slave V in the original volume, former financial executive, long-time activist, educator, mentor, and founder of several mid-Atlantic BDSM groups.

Laura Antoniou: Spelled Antonio in the original volume, now a successful BDSM novelist, outspoken activist and popular BDSM speaker.

Mitch Kessler: Aka "Sir Adam," long-time scene player, founder of NLA-NY, BDSM publisher and owner of Adam and Gillian's Sensual Whips and Toys. Married to Gerrie Blum.

Morgan Lewis HMQ: Outspoken femdom and mentor, long-time activist and board member (emeritus) at Eulenspiegel. Educator, player, group leader, and now respected elder.

Nancy Ava Miller: A vigorous proponent of femdom relationships, founder of PEP (People Exchanging Power), long-time BDSM educator and phone-sex entrepreneur.

Robin Young: Private player, best known for his foundational contributions to UseNet's alt.sex.bondage FAQ during the Internet's early days, currently helping to organize Kinky Salon Seattle

Sybil Holiday: Former burlesque star and long-time professional dominatrix, who became one of the Community's most respected educators on consensuality and power exchange in BDSM.

William Henkin: A psychologist and certified sexologist, Dr. Henkin was a trusted source on the psychology of BDSM and power relationships, both as an author and beloved therapist to many in the Bay Area BDSM community. As noted, Dr. Henkin passed away in 2014.

12 first-time interviewees

Chrissy B.: Private player, active in BDSM over 40 years, now transitioning.

Deborah Addington: Ph.D. candidate at the Graduate Theological Union, educator, ordained minister, BDSM theorist, and author of numerous books with Greenery Press.

Guy deBrownsville: Associate Member at ONYX NY (fraternal organization for men of color), Founder & Director at The Dark Lair (BDSM educational organization for people of color), and Emeritus Board Member at The Eulenspiegel Society.

Justin Tanis: Transman, educator, artist and activist, ordained minister, Managing Director at the Center for Lesbian and Gay Studies in Religion and Ministry in Berkeley, California.

Karen Kalinowski: Known professionally as *Karen The Sex Lady*, she is a kink-awareness educator, sex blogger/erotica writer, and pleasure coach.

Lolita Wolf: Long-time BDSM activist, educator, recipient of numerous awards, she blogs as "Leather Yenta" when she isn't running the Purple Passion BDSM boutique in New York City.

Nigel Cross: Private player and BDSM erotic novelist, he was formerly an officer in the US Army before becoming a computer game designer and a full time writer.

Patrick Mulcahey: Long-time BDSM activist, organizer, educator, writer, and in-demand keynote speaker. Recipient of numerous BDSM community awards, including the 2014 National Leather Association Lifetime Achievement Award.

Race Bannon: One of the most visible, vocal and respected educators, publishers and writers in the Community. Founder, Kink Aware Professionals; leader, The DSM project; bestselling BDSM author, kink columnist for the San Francisco *Bay Area Reporter*, and recipient of numerous honors and awards.

slave feyrie: Private player, in a Master/slave relationship with her (dominant) husband, she is a homemaker and, as of this writing, is an adoring mother to a beautiful, healthy baby.

slave matt: Private player, in a Mistress/slave relationship with his (dominant) wife.

Stephanie Locke: Renowned professional femdom, fetish idol, fetish movie star, former BDSM club owner, and long-time proponent of life-style female domination.

About the Authors

Dr. Gloria G. Brame

Noted sexologist, therapist and bestselling author, she is the world's foremost authority on BDSM/fetish sex.

William D. Brame

Former muleskinner and logger turned professional archaeologist, historian, and novelist, he is co-author of both volumes of *Different Loving* with his wife, Gloria.

Printed in Great Britain
by Amazon

36806646R00109